SWIMMING
IN THE
SEA OF
QI

THE TAIJI PATH TO ENERGETIC
AND SPIRITUAL AWARENESS

DENISE L. MEYER

FLOATING WORLD

For more information:
contact@floatingworldpress.com
www.floatingworldpress.com

FLOATING WORLD

ISBN 978-1-7636021-8-2
First Edition: June 2025
10 9 8 7 6 5 4 3 2 1

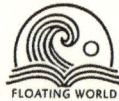

Dedicated to
Maggie Newman

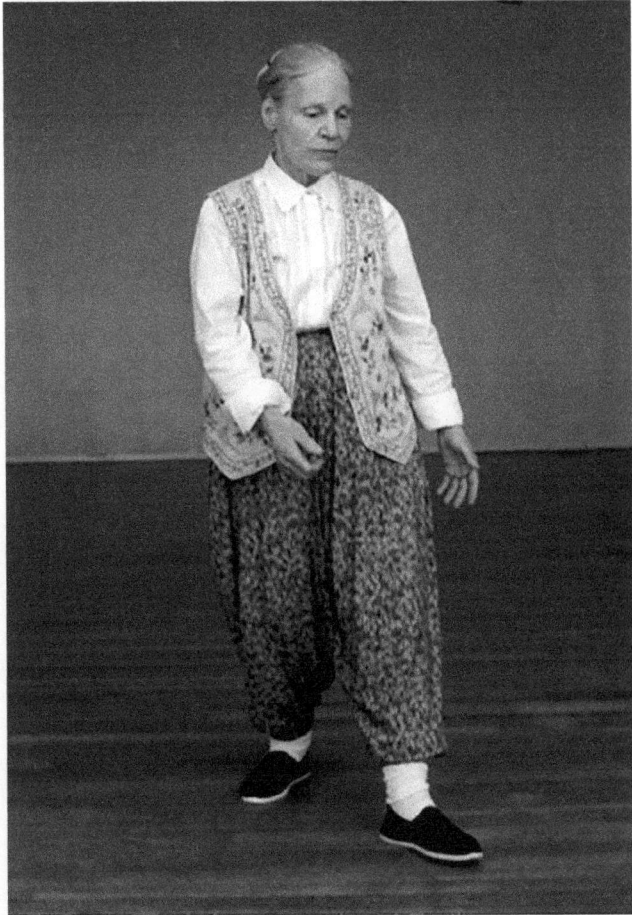

Table of Contents

Acknowledgements

This work would not have come to fruition without the many people who have contributed to my growth and insight as both a taiji practitioner and a human being. My infinite gratitude extends to:

- My taiji teachers Maggie Newman, Stephe Watson, Rob Mann, and Ken Van Sickle.

- My saintly practice partners in push hands and sword who were willing to truly work it with me: the late Michael Brody, Lynn Bywaters, Jean-Pierre Marquet, Eli Dos Reis, and Lizette Jaffrey.

- My music teachers who started my younger self on the path of taiji under the guise of saxophone: Fred L. Hemke, Lynn Jacquinn, and Ken Radnofsky.

- Willie Ruff for his consistent encouragement and cheerfulness.

- Jeff, Garret and Myles for allowing me to escape to class for these many years.

- The many people who shared their stories for this work: Linda Addison, Arthur Aronson, Lee Aichten, Carole Barber, Maria Barrett, Micaela Barrett, Rick Barrett, Sarah Behler, Steve Bennett, Lynn Bywaters, William C.C. Chen, David Chandler, Chris Chorney, David Chorney, Diana D'Angelo, Eli Del Rois, Nate Dougherty, Tom Dworetsky, Luke Faust, Roosevelt Gainey, Leyla Gulcur, Carolyn Hawkins, Jeff Higgins, Reggie Jackson, Michelle Kincade, Rick Kincade, Eleanor Lepeska, Rob Mann, Inez Martinez, Tom McKinley, Bob Messinger, Don Miller, Ming, Maggie Newman, Joseph Petrosi, Deena Reynolds, Tim Roden, Laddie Sacharko,

Scheila Scheffler, Gina Serafin, Jonathan Shear, Chenoa Siegenthaler, Libby Van Cleve, Ken Van Sickle, Bruce Walker, Stephe Watson, Cristine Wright.

- Livia Kohn, Katherine Meyer and Jonathan Bricklin who offered editorial feedback and insight; and Morgan and Catherine Buchanan of Floating World Press for bringing this book to fruition.

Introduction

How does a Western *taijiquan* player explain the onset of superhuman and mystical experiences? For many, the practice of taijiquan[1] forms, *qigong*, and push hands opens a bazaar of odd sensations—the ability to feel *qi* in one's hands, or to feel a room's energy, or to push someone twice one's weight off their feet. After a point, labeling the inexplicable *woo woo* is not good enough. As William James wrote, "Our judgements concerning the worth of things, big or little, depend on the feelings the things arouse in us" (James, 1900, p. 3).

After a few years of study those feelings in me stirred a willingness to shelve my understanding of the world, take a deep dive into the literature of nondual spiritual traditions, including classical *Daoism* and many tastes of the mystical. I began to accept the idea that manifestations of qi arise out of our alignment with the *Dao*. But metaphysical paradigms offer no concrete explanation for such daily experiences, and the most rational among us dismiss the validity of such events as spiritual experiences.

This book, by collecting stories of embodied spirituality, including mystical and psychic moments experienced by modern taiji practitioners, intends to shine light on the nondual, spiritual roots of this Daoist practice and its everlasting validity.

Although many players shy away from a spiritual view of taiji, they continue to feel good about the practice. Others are open to the suggestion that physical manifestations are possible, but simply do not have the spiritual or philosophic framework to accept this aspect

---

[1] Since most serious devotees practice a mixture of neidan practices — taijiquan, qigong, and Daoist meditation, "taiji" collectively describes these related practices in this work.

within themselves. Some simply don't recognize that the physical changes they experience might have any significance beyond the physiology of the exercise. Some describe being struck by spontaneous spiritual experiences that set off a crisis, divine revelation, or a fleeting state of grace.

The Interviews

Forty-eight generous teachers and players, ranging in age from 18 to 85, agreed to be interviewed and shared descriptions of their manifestations of qi through body, mind, spirit, as well as their deepest insights for this book. Many were friends and or acquaintances. Some were teachers I sought out; some people were referred to me. All practice taiji in the United States, and these interviews were all conducted in English. Included are 21 women and 27 men; 2 native Chinese, 1 Russian, and 1 Pole; 4 people who are Black and 1 person who is Hispanic. The average and median age was 53. The average years of taiji experience was 20; median 15. Fifteen are taiji teachers and 23 have experience with other martial arts. Included are college students, artists, musicians, writers, computer programmers, administrators, professors, social workers, retirees and taiji teachers. This work is not a quantitative study, but a collection of personal stories demonstrating the modern relevance of ancient Daoist mystical passages. Teachers of taiji are referred to using their full names. For students, I've used first name only. Sadly, in the years it has taken to write this work, a few people reached the end of their earthly journeys.

Since I've mostly tapped my personal network to access students, I have spoken with several students from within the same schools, revealing some interesting patterns. David Chandler's students had the dramatic breaking object stories. Maggie Newman's consistently evoke calmness and wisdom in their sense of mind and spirit. Rick Barrett's students have remarkable health experiences, and the attendees of his annual Taiji Alchemy weekend in Sedona report powerful mystical experiences. A number of Stephe Watson's students experienced shaking while holding poses in standing meditation.

Nevertheless, each individual's background shapes his or her sensations and interpretation of the experience; the style of taiji that they practice does not appear to fundamentally change the nature of the experience. Patterns of physical, supersensory, and psychic manifestations as well as spontaneous spiritual awakenings and a deepening sense of spirituality emerged from these accounts, becoming the organizing principle for this book.

That said, the delineations between body, mind, and spirit triggered by taiji practice quickly turn fuzzy in states of altered consciousness. Spontaneous spiritual experiences often include perceptions that can be described as either supersensory or psychic, and many of these stories could easily be classified in multiple buckets. For example, some accounts are gathered under the shamanistic umbrella because of their raw attunement to nature and those individuals' cultural roots, while others are described from a sensory perspective. My hope is not to overly objectify the nondual in this narrative, but to explore the dissolution of boundaries and form that have been part of the human experience for millennia. The experiences people have shared with me are presented alongside passages from Daoist texts, history, science, and philosophy so that we may see them through various interpretative lenses.

Nonduality

The practice of taiji along with its sister methods, yoga and meditation[2], lead us down the path of Dao—otherwise described as oneness, unity, or *nonduality*, the universe as altogether one, not two or three, not many parts, not the land of matter and myst, or subjects and objects, but nondual—One. Taiji trains us to continuously refine our perceptions and operate on increasingly subtle planes.

---

[2] Hinduism and Buddhism both arose in northern India in the fifth century BCE. Buddhism arrived in China in the third century BCE and has a long intermingling with Daoism. Today in Beijing you'll see Daoist, Buddhist and Hindu gods sitting nicely together in altars in many of the Daoist temples.

5

Probing patterns of manifestations of qi, especially those that are extrasensory or paranormal, presents an opportunity to recognize the spiritual implications of our own practice. As America's preeminent philosopher and father of psychology, William James (1842–1910), wrote:

> It is as if there were in the human consciousness a sense of reality, a feeling of objective presence, a perception of what we may call 'something there,' more deep and more general than any of the special and particular 'senses' by which the current psychology supposes existent realities to be originally revealed (James, 1902, p. 61).

Or in the words of the Daoist, Zhuangzi,

> A state in which "this" and "that" no longer find their opposites is called the hinge of the Way. When the hinge is fitted into the socket, it can respond endlessly (Watson, 2003, p. 35).

Dao and Its Engine Qi

A way that can be walked
is not The Way
A name that can be named
is not The Name

Tao is both Named and Nameless
As Nameless, it is the origin of all things
As Named, it is the mother of all things

A mind free of thought,
merged within itself,
beholds the essence of Tao
A mind filled with thought,
identified with its own perceptions,
beholds the mere forms of this world

Tao and this world seem different
but in truth they are one and the same
The only difference is in what we call them

How deep and mysterious is this unity
How profound, how great!
It is the truth beyond the truth,
the hidden within the hidden
It is the path to all wonder,
the gate to the essence of everything!

Everyone recognizes beauty
only because of ugliness
Everyone recognizes virtue
only because of sin

Life and death are born together
Difficult and easy
Long and short
High and low
all these exist together
Sound and silence blend as one
Before and after arrive as one.

— Laozi (Star, 2003, p. 26)

I nherent in taijiquan, and the related arts of Chinese calligraphy and healing, is the foundation of the Dao. Movements in the taijiquan forms illustrate its most fundamental principles. From the opening move, as you sink into your feet, your hands rise in salutation in the embodiment of Dao, or the primal emptiness. *Wu wei*, or action without doing, allows for movement without a sense of will or agency. Likewise, the interplay and interdependence of *yin* and *yang* is evident in each posture as a means of achieving balance. In that opening salutation, the sinking, or dropping of qi into the ground, is a yin movement, balanced by the hands rising in an outward yang expression.

The Daoist unity of all creatures, elements, heaven and earth is evident not only in the names of moves—such as "white crane spreads its wings" and "snake creeps down"—but in the quality of our exchanges with others as we move through space. Thus, form practice serves as a method to integrate a spiritual approach into one's life, work, and relationships. It offers a metaphysical approach to living based on the assumption of the Dao behind any activity within the universe. Other traditions may label this prime reality, life force, prana, or consciousness. Some may equate Dao with God; however, Dao does not assume any anthropomorphic properties of the guiding

8

other that dominate Christianity, Judaism, or Islam. Ralph Waldo Emerson, arguably America's first scholar of eastern philosophy and father of Transcendentalism, wrote:

> The granite is differenced in its laws only by the more or less of heat, from the river that wears it away. The river, as it flows, resembles the air that flows over it; the air resembles the light which traverses it with more subtile currents; the light resembles the heat which rides with it through Space. Each creature is only a modification of the other; the likeness in them is more than the difference, and their radical law is one and the same. A rule of one art, or a law of one organization, holds true throughout nature. So intimate is this Unity, that, it is easily seen, it lies under the undermost garment of nature, and betrays its source in Universal Spirit. For, it pervades Thought also. Every universal truth which we express in words, implies or supposes every other truth (Emerson, 2003, pp. 21–2).

This echoes *Laozi*, "Dao and this world seem different, but in truth they are one and the same," (Star, 2003, p. 14) and opens a western window toward Dao as it plays its hand through our thoughts and actions.

Or, as the Han Dynasty [206 BC–220 AD] commentator Heshang Gong describes it:

> If you can embrace the One and cause it to never leave the body, you will live forever. The One is the first product of Dao and virtue, the essential energy [qi] of Great Harmony. Therefore, we call it the One.
> The One pervades everything in the world. Heaven attains it to become clear; earth attains it to become solid; princes and kings attain it to become upright and just.

9

Entering people, it forms their mind; emerging from people, it forms their activities; spreading through people, it forms their virtue. All this is simply called the One. What it ultimately means in practice is that one makes the will one and not two (Kohn, 2016, pp. 131–2).

Taiji is, of course, both a spiritual and martial practice. At its very highest level it trains people to engage in the world from transrational states of consciousness, often making the transition from one to the other in a split second. Lawrence LeShan explains these shifts through application of a Linnaean classification of states of human consciousness and the behaviors associated with them. The spectrum he describes moves from quantitative and discrete, such as you would use balancing your monthly bills, to non-quantitative and continuous that you experience in moments of unconditional love, to the world of cosmic consciousness and satori (LeShan, 2012, p. 76). That ideal mystical state of cosmic consciousness, 'unknowing' to the Daoists, was much more commonplace to early man, who hunted, gathered, lived in caves, fully in tune with both the environment and their perceptual instincts (Kohn, 2017, p. 80-1) and presumably the proto-Daoists.

Today, most people who access the non-quantitative realms do so temporarily as they go about their lives. Perhaps they do so in a moment of push hands, joining and separating energies. For those who don't have sanctuary in the monastery, a quantitative and discrete world view is necessary to navigate the workday, perform tasks to specification and follow the rules of society. But in a flash, we switch into psychic or even cosmic worldviews. While few stay there long, these spiritual moments are fostered by taiji practices. In fact, success in the martial arts depends on one's ability to access them. That ability, to act without doing, thus dissolving subject-object boundaries, is essential to forceless martial success that is the ideal of taijiquan.

The Mysterious Qi

Fundamental to any discussion of taiji is qi, the mysterious universal energy of the Dao. Shrouded in mystery, even in the East, it is so beyond our western comprehension that most of us don't even recognize it. Daoists accept its ineffability as part of the spiritual fabric of existence. Those who have segregated their bodies and minds from spirit, don't have a platform from which to experience the phenomenon of qi, nor do they have a vocabulary for spiritual experience outside of religious dogma. Indeed, in the United States, we have a long history of intolerance toward integrated spiritual expression that shadows the ecstatic bodily manifestations demonstrated by indigenous Americans, Shakers, Quakers, and Baptists (Keeney, 2007, p. 28). Meanwhile, our culture, absorbed in object-based scientific materialism, is neither primed to recognize, nor allowed to acknowledge, manifestations of qi as they appear through taiji practice. Further complicating the situation is that qi does not express itself uniformly in each individual, and while science can measure its effects, it cannot find any "it" to study directly (Chen, 2004, 38-50).

In Verse 42 of the *Dao De Ching,* Laozi alludes to qi as the mechanism for the materialization of energy, objects, and relations:

Tao gives life to the one
The one gives life to the two
The two give life to the three
The three give life to ten thousand things

All beings support yin and embrace yang
and the interplay of these two forces fills the universe
Yet only at the still-point,
between the breathing in and the breathing out,
can one capture these two in perfect harmony.
—Laozi (Star, 2003, p. 55)

11

This suggests an awful lot goes on before the birth of yin and yang—the "two." The antecedent "The Tao gives life to one" implies a creative force or energy emanating from this source, or the means by which the Dao expresses itself. This concept was also articulated by the medieval female poet, Sun Bu-er:

Gathering the Mind

Before our body existed,
One energy was already there.
Like jade, more lustrous as it's polished,
Like gold, brighter as it's refined.
Sweep clear the ocean of birth and death,
Stay firm by the door of total mastery.
A particle at the point of open awareness,
The gentle firing is warm.

—(Cleary, 2000, pp. 430–1)

Disciple Chen Yingning's commentary on this poem strips away the metaphor:

...The "one energy" is the primal energy that is not dichotomized into opposite modes; when it becomes dichotomized, it cannot be called one energy. Confucians say, "It's being is not dual, so its creations are unfathomable." This also refers to the primal one energy. When the Old Master Lao-tzu speaks of "attaining the one," he also means getting this one energy. There is real work involved in this; it cannot be done by mere talk (Cleary, 2000, p. 404).

Although we use it widely to describe qi, the word energy is another semantic *koan*. The concept of energy has implications and shapes our thinking in ways we are often unaware of. Energy does "work" such as boiling water or driving machinery; it flows or travels between two things, and it has predictable and measurable caloric properties (LeShan, 2011). Qi is just not that tangible.

12

In a review of medical studies published in China of qigong's (which literally translates to "qi work," or "qi effort") efficacy, Kevin Chen notes that researchers found quantifiable results when measuring light, electricity, heat, sound, and magnetism as well as chemical and biological changes in the body. He concludes that despite hundreds of studies, none did much to "reveal the mechanism of qigong therapy" except for confirming that the therapeutic effects are not merely psychological but can be materialistically observed (Chen, 2004, pp. 38–50).

If qi is the purest form of life energy revealed from source, then let's presume it is Laozi's 'One.' Its manifestation is revealed through connectivity, communication, change, and movement (Rose, 2007, pp. 20–7) prior to the distinct dual perspective of yin and yang or the 'Two.'

Restated, in terms of our Greek forefathers, qi is evident in the dance between stillness and motion. Like yin and yang, these two qualities are defined in opposition to each other. One may search for the stillness in motion or the motion in stillness. And yet stillness cannot be defined as anything but the absence of motion and vice versa. Their very meanings are intertwined opposites, like the two sides of a coin; they are a unified whole.

Through today's ever popular quantum lens, one might label this zero-point energy, "the energy present in the emptiest state of space at the lowest possible energy, out of which no more energy could be removed—the closest that motion of subatomic matter ever gets to zero" (McTaggart, 2008, p. 20).

The physical nature of qi, however, remains enshrouded in the spiritual realm, hidden by the manifestation of the Two, the Three, and the Ten Thousand Things. As the vehicle of the Dao, evidence of qi is apparent, but qi itself maintains an invisible hand. David Hinton describes it as

...the generative tissue that is perennially raveling itself into the ten thousand forms, perennially unraveling itself into the ten thousand forms, perennially unraveling those forms and re-raveling itself into new forms. Here again we encounter that primal experience of time, not as linear or a metaphysical river, but as an ongoing generative moment. Or more precisely, as a place, for in this cosmology, time and space are unified into a single tissue. It is a ch'i tissue that is itself pregnant through and through; and so is itself the ongoing origin of change and transformation (Hinton, 2016, pp. 107–8).

Experientially, qi may be perceived in that blissful moment in meditation when one is in a deep unmovable state, but also feels the electric field of the body, supersensory awareness, and unlimited potential. More simply, it is sometimes evident by the presence of heat or a mass of vibrancy between one's hands when holding a standing *ichuan* position like "embrace the tree" or "small ball."

The ineffability of qi is not unique to the West. The Daoist classics protect its mystery by discouraging attempts to define qi other than to point to the Dao. "A name that can be named is not The Name" (Star, 2003, p. 55) has been interpreted by centuries of teachers as a caution. Meanwhile, the Daoist mystics historically existed on the fringes of Chinese society contributing to pedagogic tradition that favored secrecy. After imperial edicts against martial arts training in the eighteenth century (Wells, 2005, p. 2), the Buddhist Shaolin tradition modeled an ethos of clandestine pedagogical transmission that disciples of taijiquan also adopted. Given the emperor's fear of insurgents, method books were black market items shared discretely among an elite, literate class of scholars of practiced martial artists. Since personal guidance, or direct transmission, is essential to martial arts practice, written documentation has thus always been supplementary in nature. During that time, lay Buddhists taught the dharma freely and hid their martial arts. The Daoists kept both enshrouded by metaphorical and mystical verse. Furthermore, legitimate concern for harm that could be done by misuse of the practices has traditionally kept masters from open discussion with any but the most serious disciples. Post-Boxer Rebellion Chinese politics of the early 1900s turned the practice largely into a health exercise (Phillips, 2019, pp. 35–8), watering down the training for the masses but allowing the traditions to survive in the modern era. The age of the DVD and internet video has changed that self-censorship rapidly.

Concerns about open discussion are not unique to the Daoist and martial practices. Jonathan Shear, professor of philosophy, a founding editor of *The Journal of Consciousness Studies*, longtime Transcendental Meditation (TM) instructor, and a lifelong martial artist, says that most of the traditions discourage general discussion of experiences. People who do TM or Zen are taught not to talk about their experiences except in specialized contexts.

> When you're doing TM, there's no concern for the experiences at all in the actual practice. Any concern for any particular experiences means you start manipulating the meditation, and it stops working. ... What's called 'innocence' is lost. And people will start trying to get experience A, or try to avoid experience B, or start evaluating themselves. "Oh, I'm getting this and not that or this and not that." Or—Person A may have an experience. Now Person A talks to Person B, not in the presence of a trained teacher, then Person B hears the experience. Now what happens? Person A may actually be describing and putting other little things in the description, and that can distort Person A's practice. And Person B hears the experience, and then they say, "Oh, I want that," and push themselves out of shape. ...
>
> But you can talk about experiences ... in the presence of a teacher who can ward off potential confusions.

That said, Maharishi, the great spiritual leader who brought TM to the West, recognized the need for research to validate these practices for modern scientific minds and endorsed the publication of Shear's research and observations. The value of public discussion, despite the potential for distorting one's practice, is an elevated awareness of potential outcomes and a reduction of fear of the esoteric. The presentation and discussion of research results and altered states of consciousness provide a cultural context for exploring different levels of consciousness.

Taiji practice, void of any cultural context, leaves most people simply unable to recognize what is happening and without a metaphysical basis from which to process what can be startling experiences. Research results create a way to introduce such phenomenon into the minds of the scientifically and rationally thinking average American who studied Newtonian science in school and attended a dualistic church on Sunday. It brings these ancient practices back from the New Age fringe.

In the last 50 years as taiji and integrative, or alternative, healing practices have taken hold in the west, thousands of peer-reviewed studies on their efficacy in the treatment and prevention of countless diseases and symptoms of aging have reached publication. Integrative health practices have become so prevalent that the National Institutes of Health (NIH) formed the National Center for Complementary and Alternative Medicine (NCCAM) in 1991 (then the Office of Alternative Medicine). Healthcare lobbies continue to challenge the evidence, partly out of cultural resistance, and partly out of economic fear. The tide may be turning though. According to the NCCAM's 2007 study, 38.3 percent of adults (Barnes et al., 2008) in the U.S. public spent an estimated $34 billion out of pocket for the service of professional complementary and alternative medicine (CAM) providers, including $4.1 billion for yoga, taiji and qigong classes (Barnes et al., 2008). The key to CAM's effectiveness is the same for taiji, to fully embrace the nonphysical aspects of our being and psychosomatic disorders.

Unfortunately, without intellectual or cultural context, many people try a few taiji classes, admit to feeling great, then disappear, as if giving up their aches, pains, and constricted sense of self threatens their core identity. Others think something is pathologically wrong when their perception of reality is challenged by their first experience with internal energy, seeing an aura, releasing tensions, or a sudden onset of the feeling of grace. Some don't progress in their study simply because of resistance to letting go of defense mechanisms such as caving one's chest or hunching one's shoulders.

For other Westerners, spiritual dualism is so ingrained that its alternative is inconceivable. We cling to a Newtonian view of fixity a hundred years after relativity and quantum mechanics validated

16

aspects of ancient mystical spirituality. Even those engineers and physicists around us that *actually understand* quantum physics rarely allow those principles to guide their inner lives.

To live in the relative world, where linear time is undermined, and the quantum world, in which energy and matter exhibit particle-wave duality, is to soften the constructs from which we view our surroundings. Objects, even the most solid objects, are recognized as coagulated formations of energy. Beyond the mechanical understanding of how things work around us may be a more comprehensive understanding based on mystical or supersensory experience beyond the apparent realms of space and time.

After my first experience seeing my own aura, the world appeared wondrous for months. An ethereal mist swirled out of a sprouting lilac bud, visible and palpable in this transcendent state. The rock by the stream pulsed beneath me in a slow 2/4 meter. That solid hundred-year-old maple tree shading the yard became fluid as I softened; the edges between the tree and me becoming permeable. My hands as antennae, we interacted in the space between us, dancing together in a field of energy. In this nondual realm, where the tree ends and I begin becomes fuzzy, as our gaseous particulate entities merge.

Moments such as these are exquisitely powerful for those with any inclination toward nondual spirituality. Others dismiss these flashes and never move deeply into the practice. Others practice deeply and never have such experiences. To some it is terrifying. In our society, you are more likely to be considered out of your mind than in touch with spirit.

Yet Daoist literature emphasizes just such experiences, describing stages of attainment and methodology for healing, meditation, and even diet to achieve them. The ultimate achievement, immortality, is described by Livia Kohn and Chungtao Ho as a transcendent level. This level is distinguished from medical healing and longevity by the supersensory ability and mystical radiance that moves one out of the earthly realm into a spiritual co-existence with the universe and contentment with what is (Kohn, 2010, p. 75, Gajdosova, 2018, pp. 11–2). For the modern practitioner, these seemingly bizarre suprasensory events can be seen as a stepping stone to Dao.

Embodiment and the
Body, Mind, Spirit Equation

There is numinous [mind] naturally residing within;
One moment it goes, the next it comes,
And no one is able to conceive of it.
If you lose it you are inevitably disordered;
If you attain it you are inevitably well ordered.
Diligently clean out its lodging place
And its vital essence will naturally arrive.
Still your attempts to imagine and conceive of it.
Relax your efforts to reflect on and control it.
Be reverent and diligent
And its vital essence will naturally stabilize.
Grasp it and don't let go
Then the eyes and ears won't overflow
And the mind will have nothing else to seek.
When a properly aligned mind resides within you,
The myriad things will be seen in their proper
perspective.
                    —from Nei-yeh (Roth, 1999, p. 70)

The taiji road to unification plays with the body, mind, spirit equation, and how qi works its way with it. Without relaxation of the divisions between mind and body, one reinforces duality, a separation between our various aspects and Dao. These are the walls that create our sense of self, will, and separateness. As one begins to see the effects of taiji practice dissolve these boundaries, peacefulness creeps into the experience. This can be seen as a byproduct of softening physical and mental resistance, and those who acquiesce to the process can be propelled to higher levels of health and consciousness.

18

Unfortunately, "body, mind, spirit" is one of the most hackneyed phrases to evolve out of New Age spirituality in the United States. By using the phrase to sell perfumes, spa treatments, chocolate, and the latest crazes for stress relief, we distort a sacred principle. (If *only* chocolate *were* the path to enlightenment!) Commercial culture also emphasizes working on the body—striving for a quick reward of six-pack abs—and treating symptoms of stress in a merely physical manner. This approach ignores the interwoven heart-mind and spiritual components of our being, or worse, plays lip service to it. William James, in his landmark text of 1890, *The Principles of Psychology*, described "our entire feeling of spiritual activity, or what commonly passes by that name, is really a feeling of bodily activities whose exact nature is by most men overlooked" (James, 1890, p. 301).

Quantum psychologist Stephen Wolinsky starts with the premise that if spirituality is the realization that there is only one substance, "then true spirituality must include everything from emotions to thoughts and from fantasies to the physical body" (Wolinsky, 1999, p. 6).

The Paradox Known as Mind

Helpful in this process is to explore what 'mind' is. The Chinese word, *xin*, means both mind and heart, or heart-mind. This is not an easy concept for those of us raised in the "scientific" doctrine of brain supremacy. Neurologists stubbornly persist in attempting to locate the seat of consciousness in the brain despite the wealth of mystical experiences that suggest otherwise. How could an event such as precognition or an out of body experience that is characterized by one's ability to know beyond one's own personal experience, space, or time be internally generated? Such experiences suggest, rather, an ability to tap into the holographic field of consciousness with mind serving as a mechanistic muscle behind the body and its senses.

Neurocardiologists, meanwhile, lend great support to the idea of heart-mind as they unveil the electromagnetic connections between heart and brain, as well as the holographic manner in which the heart's electromagnetic field takes in frequencies of the universe through the connective tissue of the nervous system (Pearce, 2002, pp. 70–2).

Historically, the mind and brain have not been revered as they are now. The ancient Egyptians preserved all parts of the body during the mummification process except the brain, which they unceremoniously removed through the nostrils before being casting it away. The heart alone they believed to be "the center of a person's being and intelligence," (Smithsonian, 1996). Over in Greece, Aristotle and his pals located thoughts and perceptions either in the heart or the diaphragm. And in Mesoamerica, it was not just the Aztecs that thanked and appeased the gods with their most treasured organ—a freshly harvested pulsating heart—to demonstrate their humility. The ancient Daoists believed there was also a brain, or mind, in the solar plexus. Stephen Chang writes:

> We know that the entire body is operated by nerves. But whenever the subject of nerves is brought up, we invariably link in the cerebral brain while never venturing further beyond that point. The ancient Daoists went one step further by linking the nervous system to another "brain" and maintaining that that nervous center existed in the abdomen and was at least equal in importance to the cerebral brain....
>
> According to Daoism, using rational thinking to suppress true feeling is not the solution. In the *Dao Te Ching*, chapter 55, Lao-Tzu said that "in order to attain health and longevity, man must return to his infancy." The salient point is that the abdominal brain must be developed in order to recapture or maintain youth. At least both brains must be developed in balance (Chang, 1986, pp. 107–9).

In the Buddhist tradition, mind is considered a sixth sense. Thought and emotion are energies just as touch, hearing, smelling, taste, and sight are. Each pulsation of energy is there to be perceived. By focusing full attention on the breath or a koan, one quiets the power of the ego and the narrow realm it exists in, and is better able to witness what is actually transpiring in the wider mind, including arising sensation. The practices of sitting and walking meditation return one to body sensations over and over in order to better recognize the pull of mind's games. The mind, unlike any other sense, has the powerful ability to carry us off into purely intellectual realms and spin stories of self-delusion or illusion. Quieting the power of this sense is another way to create a balance from which the spiritual can be perceived.

While extensive sitting practices are an important practice for Daoists seeking the more esoteric aspects of qi manipulation and refinement (Liping, 2019, pp. 81–2), the taiji form practice brings us back into balance through body in motion. This "integration of emptiness-in-motion … is what defines the internal martial arts" (Phillips, 2019, pp. 8–22).

After one achieves a certain level of anatomical alignment and relaxation, internal energy is able to flow. The languid pace slows one's breathing while mental focus on the movements of the forms quiets the mind. In time, cultivation of that internal energy, paired with intent (*yi*), supersedes the external energies of brain and muscle that drive movement.

It is notable that the Chinese use the expression "shen, xin, yi," or "spirit, heart-mind, intent." Any focus on the body creates an impasse, merely reinforcing one's sense of self. Instead, *yi,* intent or consciousness, can be used to move you in a direction or make a limb substantial or insubstantial. The New Age mantra, body-mind-spirit, in its attempt to reintroduce balance to the equation may help over-thinkers, but it distorts and diminishes the role of *shen* and amplifies the balance of body in a way that simply is not part of the discussion in the classics. Indeed, human form is often referred to as an empty vessel which responds to spirit, qi, and intent with marionette-like action. Wang Liping's methods for internal mastery emphasize balancing original energy, transmitted energy and cosmic energy in order to transform essence into qi (Liping, 2019, p. 35). The Confucian text Wen Tzu (Han Dynasty) also emphasizes the primacy of spirit.

...The body is the house of life, energy is the basis of life, spirit is the controller of life: if one loses its position, all three are injured. Therefore, when the spirit is in the

21

lead, the body follows it, with beneficial results, when the body is in the lead the spirit follows it, with harmful results (Cleary, 1991, pp. 42–3).

Peter Wayne, a student in the Cheng Man Ching lineage and research scientist at the Harvard School of Medicine, describes the mind-brain-body relationships as a continuum.

The mind helps shape what we call the body, and the body influences what we call the mind.

This mind-body connection is referred to as the **Shen-Jing** continuum. *Shen* is generally used to characterize a person's less physical or tangible qualities, such as the thought, spirit, or emotion. ... *Jing* refers to tangible material qualities, such as the organs, flesh, and blood.

In this Chinese medical framework, you are a field of Qi, with Shen and *Jing* simpy representing different vibrational or qualitative states of energy or information. This idea is somewhat analogous to the three different energy states of water (water, ice, and steam) (Wayne and Fuerst, 2013, pp. 182–3).

Taiji Training and Wu Wei

Most of us are taught taiji under the premise that relaxation releases physical stress and allows the body, mind, and spirit to be rebalanced. That ultimately leads to better health, longevity, and changes in consciousness. Yet, for the ancient masters, to practice taiji was to strive for immortality, the highest ideal expressed in the Daoist classics.

The earth, sky, sun and moon can last forever because they follow the natural laws of the Tao. If humans are to live forever, they too must get their bodies to function according to the same laws. The two most important principles of the

22

Tao that are manifested in nature are the rise and fall and the flow and ebb of the yin and yang vapors. The rise and the fall of the vapors anchor the seasons, and their flow and ebb govern the behavior of the moon (Wong, 2000, p. 12).

Immortality has always been an unattainable goal for the average practitioner. The sages, few, though legendary, have provided inspiration and instruction just as the Buddha did for his followers and Tibetan monks do today. In all three traditions, masters strive for an inner peace cultivated by training the mind to stay with moment-to-moment awareness. To become immortal, is to stop identifying one's self with one's temporary form, and to become one with the process that never ends, allowing Dao to be the agent (Gajdosova, 2019).

The basic method in taiji is to cultivate qi. Its movement is shaped by the form's postures, informed by the five elements, qigong exercises, as well as directed meditations such as the microcosmic orbit. The physical shape of the body in proper alignment and balance will naturally lead qi to flow up the back, down the front[3], and to move in spirals[4] through the contours of the limbs. In the Yang style form, qi sinking down the legs and out through the arms is first experienced in salutation and brings awareness to the auratic sphere

---

[3] Or in reverse for women according to some sources.

[4] Spheres and spirals are ubiquitous symbols in taiji and might be interpreted as a holographic reflection of the atomic energy of the body, earth, and universe. The biologist Bruce Lipton points out that quantum physicists discovered physical atoms are made up of vortices of energy that are constantly spinning and vibrating — a "tornado-like vortex. A number infinitesimally small, dust devil-like energy vortices called quarks and photons collectively make up the structure of an atom. From far away, the atom would likely appear as a blurry sphere" (Lipton, 2005, pp. 114–15).

Both shapes are generally considered sacred due to their universality in DNA, nature and early art across civilizations. Alexandre-Emile Béguyer de Chancourtis published a period table of the elements in 1862 (arranged in a spiral on a cylinder by order of increasing with weight; his table preceded Mendelev's by seven years (Wikipedia 2019)).

around the body. The first spiral flows from that initial pivot into a ball circumscribed by the hands in the second move—peng, also known as ward off. The challenge is finding an alignment and balance that facilitates this flow.

Taiji also trains us to transcend the need to direct the body through the mind, instead allowing qi to direct movement (wu wei) while the mind (xin) takes a backseat. The condition for this transcendent state of consciousness, wu, is described variously as a state of quietude, equanimity, or more literally, "an emptiness arising from stillness." Wu is generally translated as "without" and expresses the eastern concept of emptiness, nothing, or void familiar to Zen practitioners as mu. It has also been described as "natural action" or "nonattached responsiveness" (Kohn, 2017, pp. 72–3). Wu wei bridges the spiritual and physical. In taiji practice it is used to describe movement "without action" or "without doing."

> It is important to realize, however, that *wu wei* properly refers not to what is actually happening (or not happening) in the realm of observable action but rather to the state of mind of the actor. That is, it refers not to what is or is not being done but to the phenomenological state of the doer (Slingerland, 2003, p. 7).

Wu wei is often described by taiji practitioners as the sensation of movement driven by a force that simply passes through the body rather than being the result of something one "does." This dropping of the sense of will is possible because of the absence of a sense of self. *Wu wei* is "action in which there is no bifurcation between subject and object: no awareness of an agent that is believed to do the action as being distinct from an objective action that is done" (Loy, 1985, p. 73).

While the concept is key to how a bodily activity becomes a spiritual practice, it requires a practice that emphasizes refinement and attention. Comparing taiji to other systems of nondual practice, Jonathan Shear explains:

… anything that fits the coherence of the organism can be practiced so that it comes effortlessly. It becomes suppler and suppler until it transcends itself.

In any activity, if the mind is refined enough, that can happen. I have a friend who was doing judo. When you're in the middle of it, it's like a real life and death battle. You transcend, and all of a sudden it's all gone. Everything's all gone—and look, there's the guy on the ground next to him. He would transcend in the middle of a throw. The goal of all the nondual systems, like TM, advaita, or Zen is quite explicit: it is to be in that transcendent state all the time, even while you're in intense activity. And then even further, [you] see all activity as nothing but an appearance of that transcendence.

Some argue that if you truly master martial (aka physical) technique, health and spiritual benefits of taiji will follow. Mastering may be a relative term. Those who execute from a state of *wu wei* likely have grown spiritually and have improved their health. However, the pitfall for many martial artists is resistance to softness—of tissue or ego—that prevents internal energy from harmonizing body, mind, and spirit. Regardless of one's starting point in this balancing act, one won't travel far unless the mind opens and the body relaxes into integrated attunement with spirit. Otherwise the body-self becomes an impasse with muscle leading the way rather than intent. Intent, not muscle, allows arms to be insubstantial, or yin, and thus to receive and return the more substantial yang energy.

Yi, is another Daoist term that does not translate well. While usually translated as 'intent,' Sifu Wong Kiew Kit defines it as the agent of spirit that precedes form (Kit). It has also been described as the marriage of subconscious and conscious intent that results in spontaneous physical movement. That movement is in sympathetic resonance, or harmony, with both the body and the divine, and thus results in *wu wei*, or effortless action (Wang, 2018).

In other words, when the mind quiets, the aligned body driven by *yi* moves with less and less muscular or mental work. The greater system of connective tissue and deeper consciousness slowly takes over, recalibrating the body, mind, spirit equilibrium.

Taiji Principles and Manifestations of Qi

The Quest—Ancient and Modern

For all [to practice] this Way:
You must coil, you must contract,
You must uncoil, you must expand,
You must be firm, you must be regular [in this practice].
Hold fast to this excellent [practice]; do not let go of it.
Chase away the excessive; abandon the trivial.
And when you reach its ultimate limit
You will return to the Way and its inner power.
    —from Nei-yeh (Roth, 1999, pp. 166–7)

*N**ei-yeh* (Inward Training, circa 350 BCE) is the earliest known Daoist text that prescribes methods of breathing and posture for meditation as well as exercises, diet, and sexual cultivation practices (Roth, 1999, pp. 4–18). Foundational principles of taiji practice are described in this text—contraction and expansion, the spherical shapes outlined by the path of coiling internal energy, economy of effort and movement, firmness without tension, and the need for regular practice. The taiji forms we know today, with their roots in ritual theater that knit together social cohesion alongside the temples and monasteries of ancient China, all derive basic nondual guidance from the *Nei-yeh* and subsequent texts. Later synthesis of medieval internal exercises, such as the animal frolics with theatrical portrayals of the myth of Zhang Sanfeng and combat technique, further distinguish taijiquan and its sister practices, **bagua** and **xingyi** (Phillips, 2019, pp. 24–9).

With its reliance on internal energy and integration of Daoist cosmology—in particular yin-yang and the five elements—practitioners strive for unity with Dao and as a byproduct capture its essence for martial power. Ultimately all nondual arts—taiji, yoga, meditation, tantra, shamanic journeying—are designed to awaken us to higher levels of consciousness. The end goal, enlightenment, or finding the Way, is preceded by unification of the body, breathing, and mind (Roth, 1999, pp. 166–7). The Taiji path, however, is quite different from Buddhist and Tantric methods that emphasize freedom from suffering by following strict techniques for sitting meditation. Those methods range from holding poses, sitting in stillness, drowning the self in erotic sensuality, to exploring depths of fear. Taiji, instead, emphasizes circulation of qi facilitated by movement arising from the stillness or directed circulation of qi in sitting or standing practices. Regardless, specific gestures or postures form a base, or foundation in the body that support the stillness of meditative practice (Johnson, 1996, p. 3). The continuous pursuit of these practices over thousands of years suggests a basic human need to embody spirituality.

Modern Practice

Today, people report many reasons for starting their study of taiji. Bad backs are prevalent, along with an artillery of other ailments, such as sore shoulders, fibromyalgia, chronic fatigue, or simply because it's known to be a healthy practice. A number of men, many who started studying in their teens or twenties, told me they harbor martial arts fantasies à la Bruce Lee and David Carradine. Several women began their study because of men in their lives or to meet men. Many martial artists came to taiji after extensive study and accomplishment in the more external arts such as judo, karate, or kung fu.

Ken Van Sickle, a disciple of the famous Cheng Man Ching, missed the physical contact with men that wrestling and sports offered in his youth. His martial arts journey started with karate, but after seven years and the achievement of a 3rd degree black belt, he realized the limitations of his karate teacher. I looked around to see if there was something that had more of the spiritual part that karate talked about.

27

I looked at kyudo, archery—I even looked at flower arranging and calligraphy—to find any master who was going to give me any kind of spiritual assistance, whether it was a martial art or not. Someone told me about an old Chinese master in Chinatown and I went down to see him on 211 Canal Street. I went up the stairs and saw Cheng Man Ching. After the form class there was a push hands class. I didn't know what it was then. I noticed that there were several people in that class I knew already from martial arts—kung fu, karate people, and other kinds. And he was bouncing them up in the air with effortless movements. I said, "Okay. This is something." He had both components that I was looking for. I wouldn't have to stop doing the martial part, and I could probably get the spiritual part.

For David C. it was an opportunity to carve time for himself despite his busy career and family life. While he'd always harbored fantasies about martial arts, he was also looking for a discipline that he could carry into old age without, he jokes, seeing his "arm flying across the room after having thrown a punch."

The practice quickly turned into something greater than a boy's martial arts fantasy for Nate, a recent college graduate struggling to find a career path. Poised to take a third interview for a job selling long-term care insurance, he realized, "You're selling to their fear of a terrible future, and the answer is not old age home insurance; the answer is taiji! … I really think that taiji practice and being at peace with yourself sort of kicked in."

For some, there is an equal yearning for spiritual and emotional growth. Laddie, at age 33, was in the middle of a successful career as an Army Ranger.

> I got involved in taiji when evidence and circumstances indicated to me that I was going a little bit too far in one direction. I was becoming really rigid, brittle, fixed. This is just after the men's movement wave was cresting, and we were all embracing our feminine side. I had cultivated some pretty intelligent and powerful [female] friends who discovered that there was a taiji class being offered in the Rec Department. And they said, "Come with us. This will be for you." I went. I stayed. They left.

28

Chenoa discovered taiji in college. "All I knew about it when I started was it was something that old people did." Yet before her senior year, she dropped out of school and moved across the country to study not only taiji, but also kung fu and aikido. "It feels more important to me than academic education. I feel like it's my real education."

Eli reflects, "From the time I met Sam in the late 70s when I first started doing taiji, he saved my life. I was just a young buck, doing kung fu, fighting, stuff like that. This discipline—it took me to another level."

Thirty-five years later, Eli finds that he is governed by the practice. Every day after waking, he goes outside and does qigong exercises. This is as natural to him as reaching for a morning cup of coffee.

The late Bob Messinger, who taught in Florida, had a lot of questions when he was young. The New York City school system, he says, wasn't set up for questions. Neither was his Catholic high school. He realized that all the teaching was based on separation.

I was sure that things were more connected and intertwined. I didn't have words for it then, and I'm not sure I have any real good ones now, but I knew it was so. Then the search began. I studied other religions, the occult, and got some answers, but not many. I read voraciously and that helped, but still nothing resonated.

Years later, traveling on business, a commercial for Coke came on the TV and for a brief couple of seconds there was an old Chinese gentleman doing what I later came to know as 'single whip.' "What was that?!" my mind screamed. "I must find out! The answer: taiji. Quick buy a book! No, this isn't working; order a video. Crap, that's not working either." I needed to find a teacher. Then I got a lesson in synchronicity. While having lunch one day I picked up one of those ad rags, and on page 3 there it was in bold type: Learn taiji. 10 lessons for $29.95. ... That was some 15 years ago.

A lifelong outdoorsman, Bob also sensed that his connection to nature had a religious or spiritual aspect.

> … that sense of worship and reverence found deep in the woods or on the water, or in the wonder of playing with, landing, and releasing a magnificent fish. Out there I found answers. In taijiquan I found the physical manifestation of that connection. Through taiji I came to Daoism and the knowledge that I was One all along.

While commercials on television may not be the call to attention for most of us, many people describe being attracted to the radiance or influence of someone else doing taiji.

Libby, a vivacious, tall redheaded oboist, began her study in part because her oboe teacher, the late Ronald Roseman, was involved in taiji. "He sometimes actually would stop in the middle of a lesson, he'd just put the oboe down and do a taiji move just to try to demonstrate something. Of course it flummoxed almost everybody, but I thought it was cool."

Gina, another exuberant oboist started because of Libby, although her first experiences were so powerful that she shrank in fear from the practice. In retrospect, she recognizes the deep lessons about herself and her relationship with her husband that came out of those first two-person push hands exercises.

Deena, a ballet teacher, recalls liking to watch people in New York City's Washington Square Park. She used to stop and watch her future partner practice, taken in by the slow movements.

Leyla was first drawn into taiji by the pestering of a former boyfriend. "The first week that I tried, I started feeling all these things in my body." A psychologist and a certified medical qigong practitioner, Leyla is keenly observational. She sees taiji make people more attractive as they take on qi and surrender aches, pains, and angst while generally finding greater ease being in the world.

An undefined calling to taiji is also not uncommon. Ming, an artist living in New York City, claims, "My body was yearning for this." Growing up in China, he knew about the art, saw demonstrations, and listened to discussions between his dad and his Daoist friends. Ming believed in the existence of qi but had no direct experience of it. After studying taiji, his description of his experience is typical of many. "I feel good. I really feel connected. ... You strike a pose [and] the machine is lubricated." Ming's understanding of the philosophy is to not give 100 percent. "We're brought up to give 110 percent. Relax. Don't make it happen. The philosophy is about moderation. Taiji affects attitudes. The rage in society is fueled by 110 percent effort. With taiji, attitudes relax, too."

Taiji attracts many musicians, artists, writers, dancers, and others with a strong kinesthetic sense. It speaks in a relatively familiar way to people with the internal and physical attunement that these arts also foster. Musicians, for example, routinely say taiji makes them perform better. Technique comes easier, they listen and fit into groups with ease, and can feel and train body mechanics on a subtle, interior level.

Inez, a retired women's studies professor and a lifelong student of Jungian thought, studied taiji in two periods of her life, first in her thirties and then again starting in her fifties. Of her first round, she explains that she struggled with her inferior functions, the Jungian explanation for people's strengths and weaknesses.

Carl Jung says we each have well-developed ways of perceiving the world, ways he categorizes as thinking, feeling, intuiting, and sensing. I, myself, have a well-developed thinking function. The thing is, everybody also has an inferior function. Mine happens to be sensation. .... So the first time I took taiji from Maggie Newman, I had a really hard time. I was trying to learn through ideas, and she was trying to teach primarily through sensation. I discovered after a few years that I had been doing the form all wrong—that I had never had my knees positioned so that qi could flow through me.

31

After retiring, Inez returned to Maggie Newman's classes. Having developed sensation over the years she was better able to learn through her body. As she relearned the form she was better able to apply the ideas she had heard from Maggie.

After a couple of years, I seem able to tune in to what is happening to the qi within and to practice my form accordingly. Jung also said that developing your inferior function is an important part of growing older. It helps you become more whole, more completely realized.

Although the line between personal development and spiritual practice is fuzzy, most long-term players come to recognize taiji as a spiritual practice as they synthesize the concept of *wu wei* into their movements. Learning to relate on an intimate level with this concept of "movement without doing" or "action through non-action," requires a degree of faith and trust in something besides one's own will and ability. On a practical level, taiji has lessons that are especially evident in push hands, as interaction with another provides direct feedback about one's impulses and reactions under threat. Maggie Newman explains,

Taiji is not just being able to do the form, but it has this relationship in it, which is the push hands. That can take you into a study of yourself. That makes it a spiritual development or practice instead of an ego building activity.

David Chandler, who emphasizes the shamanistic roots of taiji in his teaching, appreciates taiji as a study of transformation and the opportunities that the practice presents to experiment with change in our lives.

We look at our lives and we look at what's going on and we play our taiji; it's an experiment. The scientist in the experiment always has an effect on the experiment, so that's why they do double blinds. If you are the experimenter, you are the scientist. You are going to change that which you are experimenting on—which is you. It's a feedback loop—'Oh wow, that's interesting,'—and it takes you in a new spiral. Eventually through transformation, those series of changes, little as they are, build up until eventually people say a year or two later, "You look so much younger." [or] "You've lost weight. You look good. What are you doing? Are you in a new relationship?" Yes, with myself.

Taiji immediately became a spiritual practice for Leyla. She called it a first love. An internal energetic focus blending Daoism and Buddhism form the crux of her spiritual practice.

The key for me is that as soon as I get in touch with my body, that's when the divine comes through.

Sitting meditation, just by itself—yes, stuff will happen. Sitting, the emptying, and the stillness take me to nothingness. I'm very drawn to nothingness. But it also completely freaks me out when it takes me away from my body, particularly from this world. ... Internal martial arts, in particular, balance very well because you can do the stillness meditation and stillness practices, but at the same time, you're very heavily body oriented. You're grounding your body. All the meditative stuff is upper *chakras*, and it's letting you go off into the stratosphere. And there's something about going off into the stratosphere that feels divine. But it feels scary to me, and I feel part of my spiritual practice is to learn to be in this world.

Carole, in contrast, is very comfortable in letting go of this world. "When it feels the best to me, I'm not aware of me as much—sometimes at all. Something else happens."

Glimpsing the Numinous

The vital essence of all things
It is this that brings them to life.
It germinates the five grains below
And becomes the constellated stars above.
When flowing amid the heavens and the earth
We call it ghostly and numinous
When stored within the chests of human beings,
We call them sages.
                              —from Nei Yeh (Roth, 1999, p. 46)

For most people, attaining the benefits of taiji on any plane is not so simple as merely signing on for a six-week introductory class. Yet, sometimes, miraculous things happen to beginning students as if to simply send a message that this is worth paying attention to. Luke, for example, suffering from severe hip pain and sciatica was taken to a taiji class of Professor Cheng Man Ching in his famous Canal Street studio in New York's Chinatown in 1969 by a martial arts friend. "I sat and watched the class. I got taken to some other level; I got totally stoned just watching the class because the energy was so great. [It] just took me away."

As Luke discovered, the practice gives us the tools to transcend ordinary consciousness. While the Daoist classics typically describe this in metaphoric verse that sound like riddles to the uninitiated, this door to nonduality is palpable by all who trot in and out of taiji classes, even if one's initial motivation is to address the aches and pains of aging, injury, or to fulfill a martial arts fantasy. Over and over, we read and hear that when body, heart-mind, and spirit are integrated, we arrive at a sense of wholeness. For most people that is not a *satori* experience, but a result of regular disciplined practice over time.

Typically, the mind is overactive with doing and thinking all day. Our bodies are either neglected, as demonstrated by epidemic rates of stress and lifestyle-related ailments bankrupting our healthcare system, or the other extreme: the body is over-emphasized by adherence to the consumerist approach of the fitness, spa, and beauty industries. In one extreme, neglect of the body clogs our channels and blocks or prevents qi from passing through us. In the other, our bodies are so exalted that our heart-minds and spirit have only a vapid presence.

To integrate, according to the *Shorter Oxford English Dictionary*, is to "complete or perfect by the addition of the necessary parts" (Trumble et al., 2002). "Complete or perfect." It's hard to access that sense with a pile of housework at our elbows, family demands, the lawn to mow, and careers sucking up as much attention as we possibly can muster. The sense of something missing is often symptomatic of excessive stimulation. We already have the requisite parts—a body to carry us, a mind to help us navigate life on earth, and access to spirit driving it all. Rather than feeling we need to add something to feel whole or integrated, we need to find balance, allowing each part to shift in relation to the other.

Observing myriad taiji practitioners, from 20-year olds to 80-year olds, gradual realignments become apparent. Small shifts can manifest in logarithmic ways, in any or all of these realms, and validate this tradition. There are legions of people, a friend observed, who come to classes for a while, exclaim they've never felt better—only to drop out a few weeks later. Loss of the pain that is a somatic reflection of one's sense of self can leave one feeling empty or scared, and rather than witness their sense of self be challenged, they quit. This flight response is so innate that we're often not even aware of what we are running away from—our contracted sense of self. On the other end of the spectrum are those whose experiences of an expanded sense of self are as dramatic as accounts by Hildegard de Bingen, Eckart Tolle, and other mystics through the ages. In the middle of the road, are those who learn to recognize minute shifts in response to qi and develop in psychological and spiritual aspects—as well as in the body—that propel them to make taiji part of their life's practice.

The yen to try to describe these ineffable aspects of Dao goes back to the earliest texts. In addition to Laozi's 42nd verse of the Dao de Jing, the Heng Xian text from the Warring States Period (475–221 BCE, reconstructed from bamboo strips recovered in 1994), expounds on the nature of Dao and its agent, qi:

In the primordial state of Constancy, there is no material existence. There is simplicity, stillness, and emptiness. Simplicity is Great Simplicity; stillness is Great Stillness; emptiness is Great Emptiness. It fulfills itself without repressing itself.

Space arises. Once there is space, there is qi; once there is qi, there is material existence; once there is material existence, there is a beginning; once there is a beginning, there is the passage of time.

There is not yet Heaven and Earth; there is not yet arising, progression, emergence, or engendering. Empty, still, and as though one. Muddled and murky! All is still and homogeneous. There is not yet light, not yet teeming life.

Qi is self-generating; Constancy categorically does not engender qi. Qi is self-generating and self-arising.

The engendering of Constant Qi does not happen in isolation; there is something that takes part [in the process]. Space and Constancy are present. The same can be said of the process during which space is engendered.

Dusky and disquiet, seeking that which engenders them: difference engenders difference, returning engenders returning, divergence engenders opposition, opposition engenders divergence, and dependence engenders dependence.

[Things] seek, desiring to reproduce of their own accord. Reproduction is the process of engendering life.

Turbid qi engenders Earth; clear qi engenders Heaven. Qi is truly numinous! [Things] proliferate and engender each other, stretching to fill Heaven and Earth (Brindley et al., 2013).

As foundational as this is, such descriptions don't help practitioners understand palpable qi as experienced through the senses. Any differentiation or phenomena emerging from Dao, or One being, suggests scholar Katerina Gajdosova, is the dynamic interaction of opposites. Her interpretation of this early text suggests that when there is a boundary there is qi; and where there is qi there is something definite, yet all boundaries are temporary (Gajdosova, 2018). That dynamic interaction is, perhaps, where things become discernable to practitioners experiencing mystical changes through qigong, push hands, or form practice.

The pitfalls of focusing on qi, or its manifestations, however, are many. To name or characterize the feeling of qi objectifies it, instilling a dual subject-object perspective on a nondual reality. In *Taijiquan: Through the Western Gate*, Rick Barrett points out that when focusing on the insubstantial, its fundamental quality changes into something relatively substantial, such as the buzzy feeling many people feel in their hands, despite the fact that insubstantiality is an inherently unstable and undefinable state (Barrett, 2005, p. 38). Furthermore, such objectified feelings can create attachment that may result in its stagnation or dissipation.

And yet, as our experience becomes more dynamic, we may feel qi fill the spaces inside of our bodies and react with minds and hearts in some very profound ways. Some come to recognize the internal feeling of qi as the dancing footprint of the Dao. Even the subtlest changes in an individual's body, mind, and spirit interactions can manifest as a change in health or attitude—perhaps a lessening of pain or a change in mood. Sensing that shift indicates acceptance of a new balance. The slightest lessening of an ache can be seen as an opening to qi, whether it is triggered by an adjustment of the skeleton or by a softening of the fascia and muscles as one moves through the taiji form. Through that newly opened channel, spirit permeates. As for many of the people who have openly and generously shared their stories and understandings for this book, the journey can be profoundly miraculous as sacred threads reveal themselves through physical forms.

Daoist traditions of silence around these phenomena do not necessarily serve the modern or Western initiate having transformative experiences. Without a spiritual or philosophical basis from which to absorb and accept these gifts, one is apt to have a fear-based reaction or be close-minded about the spiritual implications whose depths can only be revealed through time and dedicated practice.

37

On the other hand, there is some basis for the code of secrecy that warrants respect. As Transcendental Meditation (TM) expert Jonathan Shear points out, the desire to have an experience like others can distort one's practice, as can interpretation of one's own experience. Longtime team teacher Laddie Sacharko puts the paradox into perspective: "I think even now, anytime I concentrate too hard on a particular awareness it goes away. It's just something you need to be open and responsive to rather than in hard pursuit of."

Laddie, remember, was an Army Ranger as a young man. He had such startling experiences early on in his practice that he knew he needed to pay attention to them. He also had welcomed the rebalancing of energies into his life. After about a year and a half of practice, he began also exploring eastern philosophies, religions, and cultures and began to develop an intensely prayerful and meditative life style, even in the midst of military decorum.

> The first thing that happened as a result of that directly, was that I was suddenly aware that my life was very seamless. Everything I needed was right at hand with no effort to look for it. Everything I wanted to do occurred with no effort to prepare for it. That's not to say that if I had to give a public speech, I didn't prepare that way, but it wasn't hard work. It was just an effortless thing that I would have to say in hindsight was very, very specifically guided—directed. From where, I don't know. But it wasn't me. Things flowed, all around me and through me and in me and out of me. And it was really good.

One principle that this statement demonstrates is a relaxing sense of self that allows one to develop the witness consciousness or "an awareness that precedes words," (Roth, 1999, p. 72). Over the course of years, daily practice becomes less about gross choreography and muscle tightness and more about how small interior or mental changes feel in both form practice and daily life. The ability to learn from perceptual inputs of the body, senses, and thought and to recognize change without becoming stuck in the mind is an important part of the taiji practice.

Martial, Health, or Spiritual?

*Positive energy can be disbursed only after it has
accumulated, negative energy can exert influence only after
it has built up. Nothing can exert influence without having
been accumulated and built up. Therefore, sages are careful
about what they accumulate.*
—(Cleary, 1991, p. 90)

One of the paradoxes of taijiquan is that it is a martial art. It is
a system for fighting, even though as an internal art it is not fraught
with visibly obvious explosive power. The power behind a taiji push
or punch can only be felt, and the uninitiated can't really see it. In fact,
to the uninitiated, a taiji demonstration may be a particularly boring
spectacle, especially when it follows a brick-breaking karate display.
Yet stories commemorating the ability of true masters to deflect a
line of strong men pushing as one, or sending a disciple flying with
the seeming effortlessness of internal energy, abound. Modern day
YouTube video not only strips away some of the esoteric mythology,
but these snippets serve to remind the rest of us of the goal of our
practice, harnessing the true power of internal energy for self-defense
and the transcendence of ordinary fear and consciousness. Of course
the teaching emphasis between martial, health, and spiritual principles
varies from teacher to teacher. And while few doubt the value of
seniors' classes geared toward health maintenance, many feel that
you are not really doing taiji unless you are martially effective. As
instructor Joseph Petrosi says, "If you are doing the martial right,
the rest comes."

The downside of the martial attitude is a reliance on power and
not truly developing yin, as seen through softness of the push and
willingness to simply neutralize a situation. There is no doubt that
players who feel like solid stone pillars are using qi and **root** rather
than muscle, but the effortless feather-like push or disappearance of
mass that Cheng Man Ching's students describe of him is missing. The
classic push hands verbal standoff is accusing your partner of using

muscle, rather than qi. Not only is it difficult to distinguish between a forceful yang energy and pure muscle, it is confoundingly difficult to train oneself to stay soft while encountering force. Nevertheless, on the receiving side, being uprooted rather than shoved is easy to distinguish.

On the other hand, some teachers emphasize health to the detriment of good technique as the execution of a proper push or shoulder strike is irrelevant to them. Attention to learning a move martially would ultimately strengthen the healing aspects of their taiji since the martial doesn't work without good alignment, proper balance, and root. Moreover, those who don't embrace push hands practice, and therefore, the martial aspect, often are lacking strong root. One can feel the flow of qi without it, albeit with some risk of *kundalini* psychosis. Root provides both an emotional and physical safety net that allows one to practice with another person within the intimate arena of push hands.

That said, there does seem to be consensus that spiritual development can flow from either emphasis. The opening of channels leads to a palpable flow of qi, moment to moment concentrated awareness, and the consequent sense of wellbeing—if not occasional euphoria.

Bob Messinger recognized that the martial practice goes beyond defense against physical attack but also provides protection on the spiritual and mental levels.

> ... being a Daoist martial art, it has to meet certain criteria: That it protects the body at every level—spiritually, physically, mentally. That it will protect, not only from invasion or attack by human beings, but attack by almost anything—pressures, stress, animals in the wild, whatever. As it's come up through history, it's been found to have a profound effect on certain aspects of health. It strengthens the immune system and gives an immediate sense of balance and an increase in the body's physical balance. It brings about a connection both to earth and also to heaven as you practice.

As we established earlier, spiritual essence can be recognized through bodily sensation, and physical practices can be refined to where the mind shifts into higher levels of consciousness. However, the meeting of martial and spiritual also takes place in the realm of heart-mind, where one learns to settle one's emotions and face fear—fear of relationships, fear of assault, fear of the future, fear of death. Ken van Sickle explains:

> In order to experience or evolve spiritually, a person has to first pass many obstacles. Those obstacles are fear and desire. Fear and desire which can come in many forms— ambition, fear of death, many things get in the way of our spirituality. The process of taiji, first as an exercise, just an exercise, and then a social interaction, and then martial art is to keep you—even if you're being attacked—completely unafraid, "unangry", and just there in a calm accepting state. … Then, taiji, because it also is meditation in movement, allows you to start to contact, and come into contact … and leaves you open to more spiritual undertaking.

Reflecting on a workout between two taiji sword fencers we'd observed together the week prior, he noted:

> The fact that a sixty-year old handicapped woman can beat a young, very strong athletic and fairly accomplished man with a sword proves the axiom that taiji is a martial art that uses the energy of the other person, and you effortlessly return that energy to them. When it is done well, following those principles works. It is very difficult for people to do it well and follow that principle because the ego gets caught up and starts wrestling and struggling. Struggling—there's either effortlessness or struggling. As you start to struggle, you're not doing taiji anymore.

That acceptance of what is transpiring, is, in essence, what the martial training is about. The training leads one to overcome the fear that readily arises from the threat of letting someone get intimately close. The threat of intimacy is both emotional and physical, and, of course, a punch to the face, a kick to the groin, or shove to the body, is an insult to the ego. Acceptance without fear, allowing events to unfold with a calm response, takes a deep sense of peace and transcendence over one's animal instincts. This ideally grows to an acceptance beyond the martial sphere into daily encounters and personal relationships. Cheng Man Ching is shown on video deflecting a line of ten men pushing against him and also sending student after student flying through the air. In teaching push hands, says Maggie Newman, he talked about not entering conflict, instead focusing on technique and strategy so that you did not set yourself up.

> Basically he got the big picture, which was don't go against them. He was able to not force his opponent. *Not force his opponent*—that's a high skill. It was said that he could do that after he had a dream that he had no arms, so somehow, he discovered how not to use the force of his arms ... He was able to demonstrate that he didn't go against what was happening, but he went *with* what was happening.

That moment-to-moment awareness, willingness to merely neutralize an incoming force, and acceptance of what is unfolding without emotional reaction, is indicative of a high degree of spiritual attainment. Taiji student and philosopher, Jonathan Bricklin, writes:

> Given that the contractile emotions of anger and fear cannot be experienced in one-pointed *sciousness*, it comes as no surprise that they are absent from accounts of enlightened persons, such as the Buddha. ... While both anger and fear are commonly believed to focus attention, they are, in fact, always a sign that attention is, instead, distracted. As every accomplished martial artist knows, neither anger nor fear facilitates the moment-to-moment awareness required for self-defense. Indeed, the greater the absorption in the precise movement of, say, a fist coming towards you, rather than in

any feeling you might have about it, the greater the chance of avoiding it. To those for whom being in the moment is not a wish but a realization, adrenaline is not needed to make them more alert (Bricklin, 2007, p. 69).

The progression toward moment-to-moment awareness, however, is not obvious or easy. The vast majority get glimpses and grow towards it in fits and spurts. For many it is an unintended result stumbled into. Bob Messenger, for example, was not initially attracted to taiji as a spiritual practice, although that very quickly became intertwined with the martial, as the connection to spirit was raised for him through physicality.

You can understand the connection more deeply because you have that physical connection. I didn't have a practice of study that did that. Meditations and fishing and sitting in the woods and listening and watching were my only practice for that. So this has become, at least, a physical manifestation of my spiritual beliefs, but only through study of it as a martial art. If you study it solely for health, I don't think spiritual transformation can take place. I think maybe partially it can, but without at least a deep understanding of the internal purpose of the motion, not the external, I don't think that you could truly get as much out of it as you can if you do study it completely.

For others, the taijiquan forms are a tool for meditation and personal development or a way to calm the mind. Thirty-two years into his study Tom M. recognizes the martial applications and health applications, but his interest is in perfection of the form. "Maggie [Newman] described taiji being a kind of movement koan, like a zen koan, and it's something you constantly try to perfect or try to understand and use to move yourself along."

Looking at the practice from an integrated view of personal development on all levels, martial artist, teacher, and writer Don Miller observed a number of martial artists who made very rapid progress in certain aspects through taiji and related arts and got a lot of power before their personal development caught up with their energetic or martial development.

I have a concept of mastery that is uniform—which is to say, that there are physical skills, psychological skills, spiritual skills, and emotional skills, and it's not mastery if you throw someone into the trees and go home and kick the cat.

To me, the notion of mastery is consistent across all aspects of someone's life. If you're really practicing all aspects of the art, it will develop you evenly. But what happens, particularly when you're younger, is you go for the power parts of the art, and they're available. And you get very powerful, but you don't necessarily get wise. You look at someone like Cheng Man Ching; it seems like his development was pretty even, as well as the fact that he was not only a master of taiji, but also of medicine and calligraphy and philosophy and brush painting, and a whole lot of other things. He was well-rounded and not carried away with his taiji prowess.

While many people describe their taiji practice as a letting go of sensory boundaries and physical constraints, Maggie Newman sees taiji's structure in movement as a metaphor for living. Like the writer who finds freedom of the pen only under the constraint of a deadline, the principles of the taiji form provide boundaries from which to learn to operate.

We all have different tendencies in our personalities. If I'm left to my own means, everything is so interesting that I will follow like a child in a candy store. ...

As a child doing writing exercises—making O's—I could not stay on the page. If I'm left to my own devices, I will get too big. Structure stops me when I want to do a gesture that's all out—but it is more like a frame of reference that

44

tells me where I am. It's also about being happy, finding some happiness and comfort in the external form that you've been given.

In the beginning, so that you experience some principles of the universe, which has balance, we use the form externally. And that experience—that balance in its specific shape—is given from the outside. If I can find and make myself at home there ... *It's like going through discipline to freedom.*

That's the way I think about the form or any kind of form whether it's Kabuki form, a dance form, or whether its taiji. First, there's a certain form there because they discovered some principles. They imitated the principles in the universe of our natural movements. And then people who are uncoordinated and unbalanced in their natural walking, or whatever, can do this form, and they learn something about a natural kind of balance and flow that serves them in their life.

That balance may be achieved on a physical level by learning to not over-extend the knee shifting into a bow stance, or to keep a punch connected to one's center of gravity by not overextending. On the mind level, balance may be achieved by focusing on the body as one moves through the form, or on the cause and effect, or move and response, that are pursued in push hands. The spiritual result we aspire to with these shifting dynamics is a sense of peace with our existence in the world.

Root

The heavy is the root of the light.
The unmoved is the source of all movement.

Thus the Master travels all day
without leaving home.

However splendid the views,
she stays serenely in herself.

Why should the lord of the country
flit about like a fool?
If you let yourself be blown to and fro,
you lose touch with your root.
If you let restlessness move you,
you lose touch with who you are.
                    —Laozi (Mitchell, 1999, p. 27)

When we talk about balance in taiji, we draw on two key elements. First are the mechanical skills that keep the body within its center of gravity by not overextending, reaching, or leaning. Second is the principle of root or one's relationship to the ground. This concept is most often illustrated by analogy to a tree, whose health and stability are dependent on its growth deep into the earth to balance the reach of its branches. Taiji forms first initiate relationship to the ground in the opening salutation where we establish ourselves as a bridge between heaven and earth. In that move we have the capacity to energetically connect to qi in its many expressed permutations. In the spine, we establish our alignment and allow the qi to sink through the legs to, paradoxically, raise the hands. In our minds we shift our attention into the practice and attune to whatever our focus is for the session. In spirit, we enter into a position of offering and receiving qi to and from the greater universe.

These forms also create connections to root that people may otherwise be lacking by their very nature. A flighty person we say needs grounding. A pedant lacks the lightness of the spirit beyond mind. Only by tapping into both heaven and earth does balance through every action or moment become plausible. Root, or that connection between heaven and earth, keeps us in our bodies and in this world, at the same time that it allows us to expand beyond the boundaries of the body into the supernormal or mystical realms. The body, meanwhile, becomes a conduit for this puppetry.

46

Many practitioners work hard to develop root through rigorous standing meditation practices or neigong (energy gathering exercises). William Chen's famous Three Nails approach optimizes the way the foot, specifically three energetic meridian points in the sole of the foot, touches the ground. Other teachers claim one should focus on the bubbling well point (the point at the front of the arch below the middle toe mounds) as it makes contact with the ground; Rick Barrett demonstrates the effectiveness of pointing the index finger as a way to make the body energetically coherent. A range of visual images also can be effective, such as visualizing tree roots, the core of the earth, being buried down to one's waist, etc. In push hands, however, deep connection to ground that is static can easily be challenged by a skilled player capable of "uprooting" dead weight. Even in rooting, one needs balance and buoyancy. To stubbornly try to connect to ground and bounce off an opponent instead of engaging in a conversation by neutralizing incoming energy can be as limiting as using muscle force to slam him or her into a wall.

True root reflects the ability to adjust your relationship to gravity, neutralize incoming forces, and hide your center through the balance, relaxation, and surrender of the body (song). It can be as light as a feather—as demonstrated by Cheng Man Ching—or solid as an iron boulder. Root is the great equalizer that allows a five-foot female to send a six-foot male flying in push hands.

"People often put relaxation [song] as the primary principle in taiji and root as one of the subsequent ones," says Don Miller,

> [I]n my experience, while they're certainly interrelated as all the taiji principles are, if you don't have root, you can't relax. Your system senses its vulnerability in asking it to give up its armor, and its reliance upon muscular strength and power and external physicality. It's really unfair to ask yourself to do that until you have an alternate pattern that will keep you safe, and your system knows that.

Root has been a deep focus of Don's practice over the years. He relates an experience with colleague Rick Barrett some years ago in Manhattan's Washington Square Park playing what they called "elephant wrestling," in which both people stand upright with feet parallel facing each other. Don had been practicing with the image of connecting his root all the way to the molten core of the earth via a cable. Normally Rick would have been able to move Don in this game. But that day, Don was immovable. To Don, that was an objective validation of what he was feeling. "It's what Uncle Bill [Willem De Thouars], my martial arts teacher, describes as "internal cultivation and external manifestation," he said.

Root's safety net is not only key to relaxation and push hands prowess, but also to mental safety within energetic spiritual practices. The late Roosevelt (Rosie) Gainey, a Daoist priest from Brooklyn, primarily taught proper body function through posture and breathing to anchor to qi in a safe way. Starting with what he called the Three Presses—the feet into the ground, the sitz bones dropping, and the neck pressing back or elongating—the skeletal alignment straightens into a c-shape facilitating the energetic pass up the spine while increasing one's breathing capacity. This alignment is key to staying in touch with the earth and preventing kundalini psychosis triggered by unbalanced energy in the upper dantien or third eye.

See, there's three dantiens. The lower, the middle, and the upper. This [the middle] one you can mess with a little bit, but this is the seat of emotional cleansing. But you best not mess with the third eye. You ever seen anybody who really meditates a whole lot? And you look in their eyes? Don't they look scared and ready to [take] flight? They're ready to run to the mountains. They all got to get into the monastery. They went from this world.

... I teach that you're like a hula-hoop. That's the shape of your body. And it's full of energy everywhere at once. So when one part moves, every part moves. I found it's been quite spiritual for people to move energy and break up points one after another. ... You do everything gradually. Gradually you'll be awake at the same time. Safe, safe, safe. You get called, your mind goes over there as you go over there, energy moves out of that midpoint.

You can create a problem for yourself—a sensory problem, where you become hypersensitive to things. When people's energy is insane, you'll be watching TV and see a commercial and cry at the commercial. They're unbalanced. The slightest thing could upset you, drive you crazy. ... I've got a lot of yoga people that are terrified of doing yoga anymore, because of what it did to them mentally. [More on kundalini psychosis later.]

David Chandler, a taiji and acting teacher, talks about root and alignment as it enhances access to one's personal power in daily life.

When someone is simply standing, and they lock their knees, shoulders being up, the tendency is for them to lose their energy, and they're uprootable. They're really easy to knock over. ... In a sense it's where evolution has taken us: out of the trees and back on the ground. When we get frightened, our shoulders go up. Sometimes fear grips us and we go completely still. That might save us, being totally quiet and not moving. "It might not see us, they'll eat something else." Or we fight. Fight, flight, run away. Scream. Make the big noise.

So to access your power you drop those shoulders, opening the body. For instance, you sink your qi. You drop your chest, you create a dove's egg under each arm. Drop the tailbone; you sink the sacrum; bend the knees. The knees are slightly bent. Now you access the earth energy with your mind—we call it 'bank line taiji' in our school—where you stand in line someplace and people will lock their bodies up and they won't have any power. They're stressed out thinking, "This line is too long."

Instead, settle down in those circumstances. Instead of being in a situation where they're locking their knees and cutting the circulation off, open their knees, they're suddenly now not in the joints where they can wear out. They're now

49

in their thighs and now in their body in a whole way. Their spine is aligned. In that spinal alignment you can access the energy from the earth.

The earth is a giant magnet. So when you sit into your body in this fashion, you access the power of the earth. So you also begin to work with gravity instead of against it. Working with gravity, you have power. Gravity is power. And so when you have that kind of alignment, and you're sinking, you're now aware. Your awareness has grown. You're transcending this body to a larger arena of space. And so, what that does is initiate a first level of response. When you put your spine in this kind of alignment, the tailbone tucked and lengthening up, what we call the c-shape of the spine instead of the s-shape. [This makes] a connection for the brain that allows us to not be triggered from a place of reaction, but from a place of response. So your most primitive responsive animal is keyed in. The reptilian portion of the brain is ready to go. Have you even tried to catch a lizard or catch a snake? They're fast. They're responsive. They're not reactive. … You'll be in readiness state. So your animal is prepared. And your higher nature has a leash on the animal.

Root then is a multipurpose asset. It grounds us physically and mentally; it is a safety mechanism; it is a foundation for personal development; and it allows us to operate in a state of transcendence regardless of whether our focus is in the martial art, health, or meditative aspect of the practice. Root also quickly becomes a benchmark for how we judge teachers, push hands players, and even how attractive one appears doing a form in the park. Technique, relaxation, and root find equilibrium; and qi passing through radiates around the individual just as new life that shines through a pregnant woman.

Push Hands

True power, then, emanates from consciousness itself;
what we see is a visible manifestation of the invisible.

—David Hawkins (Hawkins, 2002, p. 134)

Tui Shou, or push hands, sometimes called sensing hands, is a part of the martial tradition that turns taiji into life's laboratory. It is a practical method for learning to express the inner power, *te* (Roth, 1999, p. 145), that is cultivated through form practice and it is also mirrored back to you by a partner. As the c. 100 BCE text Wen-Tzu states,

> The learning of those who listen with their ears is in the surface of their skin. The learning of those who listen with their minds is in their flesh and muscles. The learning of those who listen with their spirits is in their bones and marrow (Cleary, 1991, p. 62).

Through two-person interactions one's limitations, emotional patterns, habits of response, and sense of separation are brought to the surface. Once that window opens, it is hard not to also see these patterns in one's personal life—whether navigating the stormy waters of independence-hungry teenagers or a difficult boss. Developing the inner calm that allows a response rather than a reaction to these lessons is part of the journey. In push hands, the difference between reacting and responding can be the difference between a shove and a press; and push hands practice, like life, offers a great deal of repetition from which to gain skill.

The four-move form that many practice, peng-lu-chi-an (ward off, rollback, press, push) reinforces the principle that any outward push is preceded by a neutralization or allowing an opponent's energy in. This too, is a reflection of ancient ideals:

To contract is a means of seeking expansion, to bend is a way of seeking straightness. To contract an inch to expand a foot, or bend the small to straighten the great, are things that superior people do. —Wen-Tzu (Cleary, 1991, p. 166)

Sparring without this interplay of sending and receiving is ineffective and instantly turns into a wrestling match. Those who can operate from a place of higher consciousness, even when under threat, succeed. It is a supreme test of one's ability to harmonize yin and yang and maintain a nondual state of consciousness.

When focused on sensing a partner's energy in such a state, the game softens and time slows down. The realization years ago, that I could know the essence of a person within minutes of playing push hands was a profound and difficult development, especially when that truth is one you've missed through a long relationship. On the other hand, it is a wonderful way to make friends with people that you would never have connected with otherwise and to appreciate our interconnectedness.

Oftentimes the energetic interaction with another, like a good healing session, can trigger the exhilarating feeling of dancing with qi. One divorcée told me that the interaction with male energy kept her from going crazy in the years when she was not in a relationship.

Tom D. recalls his days in Cheng Man Ching's studio when every now and then the Professor would look up and say "good push." He said you can hear a good push; it sounds like a pop. Scuffling, feet sliding, or grunts are indicative of a bad push. Tom took from him that if you just treat this like a game, the doors of understanding are closed to you forever. That does not mean it requires devoted attention to martial applications, but rather that it's about the natural order of things.

Push hands allows me to face the issue of death in my life. I mean that's what martial arts are about, right? They're about preparing for that moment. ... They're not dancing and looking good. They're about being centered under the maximum pressure a living being can be under, which is:

52

You're going to die. If you're not thinking like that, your practice is hollow, in my opinion.

Preparing for the moment that separates emptiness and fullness—life and death—gives you the calm in a crisis, whether it's a car crash or fight, without which, none of your techniques are going to work. The difference between Electric Louis [a boxer] and a normal civilian wasn't that he was big and strong and tough and mean. It was that he didn't get tense. His energy didn't come up out of his root because he was getting into a fight. He settled down. He hit the zone. He got calm. That's the difference between a prizefighter and a civilian. That's the difference between an athlete or an actor, and a civilian. That's what we're practicing here.

The ability to listen to people is one of the greatest benefits that Tom attributes to his taiji practice. At work or at home, the difference between physical listening and aural listening disintegrate. By dropping fear and pride from the interaction and becoming more of a neutralizing person, he has grown.

One of the things that is important to acknowledge, in any practice, is that if you have to be rigid to be perfect, you've set up yet another problem. So, yes, I lose my temper; I do have anger; I do have issues, they do come up. But when they do, and the Karma returns to me, I understand it; that's a learning moment.

Philosopher Jonathan Bricklin, who has practiced taiji for three decades, writes that the contracted emotion, anger, represents a contracted sense of self. "… [T]hat anger is always a lesson; and to the degree that we stay angry we haven't learned it" (Bricklin, 2016, p. 154).

Learning lessons from anger, says Tom D., leads to a change in alignment both internally and to the outside world, including to people and events in one's past.

I think that taiji gave me the confidence to appreciate the humanity in people no matter how crazy they are. And that projects to them. I mean most people just want to be treated with respect. They want to be acknowledged, recognized as people. Whether they are beggars on the street or… Nobel Laureates—it doesn't really matter.

On a physical level, Lynn describes a pattern emerging from push hands of one hand getting hot while the other turns stone cold. Sometimes she feels what she describes as a "not unpleasant" prickly sensation around her wrists and up her arms. With one particular advanced partner who played with the intent of sending qi through to particular *Dim Mak* points, she described lasers of energy shooting through her. She credits them with obliterating a benign ovarian cyst. When I was the recipient of that technique, a wave of nausea overtook me as the qi flowed up my arm and into the kidney area.

Recalling a demonstration for police officers, instructor Joseph Petrosi describes a *big* guy following him around the room all afternoon, demanding,

"How did you do that?" I said, "Your qi flows." We always taught that qi is like an army inside you. If you get hit, your qi rushes to that point to protect it. … Most of the army goes to help it and the rest of it goes back to where it should be. So in taiji we're taught to strike to bring the qi somewhere and then strike again where we know it's not.

On the opposite end of the spectrum, Maggie Newman describes the gentleness behind a push from Cheng Man Ching as not feeling invasive, but safe and exciting. "It didn't feel like bone on bone. It didn't feel like he was pushing you."

Ken Van Sickle also recalls that when Professor Ching pushed you, it didn't feel like a push from 99 percent of people.

Instead of feeling a point of being pushed at, it was like a wave; an ultra wave that picks you up so you don't know where the push is coming from. It's just one big movement. You get lifted off the ground and drawn back. Defending against a push, you couldn't find him. He was in the clothes somewhere but you couldn't find where. And then when you got all the way back and you were overextended as you began to retreat, all of a sudden there was something very powerful there. … He'd catch you on the retreat and that's why you go so far.

Micaela describes push hands as another way of talking, a different way to communicate with people, and Gina, who discovered taiji as a graduate student with her husband, also learned to listen in a different way. In fact, after a couple of sessions she became scared by what emerged about them as a couple.

I realized in terms of energy that there were control issues. I felt that during the push hands Stan wasn't listening to me. And that he was dominating the exercise. Back then, I did what I did back then, which was retreat. You know, now I can look back at it and realize that I wasn't bringing my energy up to match him. Whenever I tried to match, it didn't feel right. It felt like he wasn't responding. It was an eye opening experience because the exercise, for me, revealed that there were issues in our relationship—control issues.

Describing the evolution of her push hands practice over the course of thirty years, Maria recalls gaining the ability to observe when the energy or emotion she was feeling was not hers. Maria was always somewhat of an empathic psychic. Although she'd never cultivated her abilities, she would frequently start to feel sad or depressed for no apparent reason, especially on the subway. After studying taiji, she recognized that it was not her energy causing these emotions, but one that she'd in some way touched or taken in. Learning to expand her awareness and look around she could often discover the source.

With more experience, she also began to be able to apply her push hands lessons at work. Rather than pushing away when feeling stress or dealing with conflict, she learned to channel the energy or move it in another direction rather than rigging up against it, even in a verbal exchange. She describes this as living from a more internal point of view where you step back from the drama and work with the energies passing through the body.

For Arthur, push hands opened up the wondrous, and as a result it became the central part of his taiji practice. He discovered that by relaxing and finding the flow, he could do things that as a relatively small man, he couldn't otherwise do—defend himself or move somebody. Recognizing this paradox,

Everything else became incidental because that was a training ground, a real training ground for making stuff that was flights of whimsy, or vague, abstract ideas, real. I had repeated experiences of relaxing and having power. There was a partner that was trying to push me over, and I became more and more successful in avoiding that result the more I calmed down, adopted a posture and used a very elementary technique of pointing [taught by Rick Barrett]. When that stuff started working it was a bit on the miraculous side.

Mind Body Connections
and Wellness

Health and Healing

If people can be aligned and tranquil,
Their skin will be ample and smooth,
Their ears and eyes will be acute and clear,
Their muscles will be supple and their bones will be strong.
They will then be able to hold up the great Circle [of the Heavens]
And tread firmly over the Great Square [of the earth].
They will mirror things with great purity.
And will perceive things with great clarity.
Reverently be aware [of the Way] and do not waver,
And you will daily renew your inner power,
Thoroughly understand all under the heavens,
And exhaust everything within the Four Directions.
To reverently bring forth the effulgence [of the Way]:
This is called "inward attainment."
If you do this but fail to return to it,
This will cause a wavering in your vitality.

—from Nei-yeh (Roth, 1999, p. 76)

P hysical unity with the Dao allows its engine, qi, to work through the body, disassembling the physical and mental fortresses that reinforce the illusion of self. That change in relationship, not only to one's own self but to others, is key to martial arts. Frequently, the changes that first get the attention of adult students, however, are changes in health or a healing.

Desire for improved health is, perhaps, the easiest point of entry into the practice. To have the body functioning in optimal condition without being bound by aches and pains can open one's eyes to the miraculous. "One of our main responsibilities as human beings is to take care of the body that we're in," offers Ken Van Sickle, who at age 75 stands perfectly erect in the body of a far younger man. Still, he likes Cheng Man Ching's plug for the martial aspect as well: "Yoga is great, but what if someone tries to knock you off your cushion?"

Discussion of health benefits naturally leads to the image of taiji classes geared to older people. From China we see photos of hundreds practicing in the parks in the morning, and in the U.S. classes in senior centers abound. "Seniors" has misleading connotations for longtime practitioners like Maggie Newman, who at 85, and Ken van Sickle at 75, belie their ages.

At age 90, my grandfather's arthritis—most visible in the gnarled hands and swollen knuckles that reflected a lifetime of hard work— presented a serious quality of life issue. He had a few taiji lessons and practiced with the teacher's videotape, and felt immediate relief from pain. This is a typical response, and research shows that the mere introduction of qi rejuvenates the body's microsystems of bones, sinews, and fluids[5]. That results in increased circulation and a lessening of pain as the joints are lubricated, and inflammation and blockages give way.

With my grandfather in mind, I visited a class offered at a local senior center. None of these elders were concerned with martial prowess and none had started taiji before their late sixties or seventies. Most exhibited some signs of the inevitable physical and mental deterioration of age. Their enthusiasm and observations reinforce the idea that it is not about achievement; it is about process. Just showing up and doing it, however many modifications necessary, can lead to palpable results. Joining the late Bruce Walker's class for two weeks, I was also surprised at what a workout I got. He didn't

---

[5] A 2016 Pubmed search of meta-analysis studies on taiji and arthritis shows largely positive effects even from limited practice (Astin et al., 2003, Lee et al., 2007, Reid et al., 2008, Hall et al., 2009, Iwamoto et al., 2010, Schieir et al., 2010, Bennell and Hinman, 2011, Yan et al., 2013, Lauche et al., 2013).

expect his seniors to be entering competitions, but they stuck with him through a rigorous set of esoteric kungfu exercises and a Yang style long form. In fact, the content of the workout was no different from that of his studio class filled with strapping young men and women in the prime of life, except for a few modifications for those using wheelchairs and walkers. Comments from Bruce's seniors reflect myriad health improvements:

- "It feels good. The stretching and stuff relaxes me."
- "I go home and I just want to lay down because I'm so relaxed from it."
- "More stamina."
- "Much better balance."
- "It's helping me with bending."
- "My blood pressure is right in the middle."
- "I haven't gotten a cold, knock on wood, in two years since I've been doing this."
- "I haven't gotten a cold, and I used to have asthma."
- "If you miss a week, you really feel terrible."
- "All the aches and pains go [away]. I think mentally you're more alert. You have a better outlook."

One woman had lost her vision in recent years. She joined the class to help herself deal with the anxiety and tensions that blindness added to her life. But she also gained a level of confidence that empowered her to start taking the bus by herself, regaining the freedom and independence she'd sacrificed with the loss of her eyesight.

Another woman acknowledges the calming effects of the practice, saying "We in this world are generally rushing around, and [taiji] makes you slow down. ... so your interactions with people become better."

The late Reggie Jackson, a taiji player and teacher for 30 years, in his late 70s looked like he was 55 with smooth soft skin, erect bearing and a spring in his step. It was a shock when prostate cancer took hold and metastasized to his spine, rendering him paralyzed from the waist down. At the nursing home, Reggie, surrounded by books on taiji, practiced his form and the microcosmic orbit from his bed and wheelchair. When interviewed six weeks before his death, he still had good color, and loved to talk about taiji. He proudly showed me how he could lift his leg—just a hint—doing the form in his wheelchair. Even while his PSA levels were soaring, until the last few weeks, he was not overtly showing signs of pain or sickness. Approaching his eightieth birthday, he simply wasn't a 'senior,' he was cracking jokes and living a mentally stimulating life from his half of the nursing home room.

On a more benign level, Rick Barrett gained three inches in height doing taiji all these years. In the first seven years of my practice, I, too, gained ¾ of an inch in height[6]. Since I started practicing in my thirties the idea offered that I'd actually grown bone was laughable. While some of that height is likely postural improvement, a portion of that height Rick speculates comes from an increase in the synovial fluid cushioning the vertebrae.

Maria describes how the form began to be a barometer for how things were going because she could tell where her tensions were. Several women describe easy menopause with minimal hot flashes and none of the extreme symptoms bemoaned by so many. Roosevelt Gainey laughingly tells of several women who want to kill him because they started menstruating again after balancing their hormones by walking the bagua circle, a phenomenon also experienced by a taiji classmate as she approached her sixtieth birthday.

Observations of health changes ring true for the younger population as well, and those changes are also just as likely to be emotional as physical. Bruce Walker's studio was near a mental health facility. A lot of his students suffered emotionally from abuse, sexual or physical, and were as he described, "frozen in fear. ... I've had people tell me that they feel much more confident and powerful from

---

[6] While I have not found research on this phenomenon, per se, there are many studies that demonstrate that even short-term practice can improve balance, circulation, the fascia, etc. Taiji is also one of the forms of exercise often recommended to prevent osteoporosis in the elderly.

taiji, and they're more able to get out and talk to people."

Luke, remembering his earliest days in taiji recalls,

> I was living on the Lower East Side at the time and …
> I had mosquitoes in the apartment. I started waking up in the
> morning and the wall next to my bed would be dotted with
> dead mosquitoes. I was killing them in my sleep, and I knew
> that was the taiji at work with my reflexes getting faster.

Suffering chronic knee pain from his high school lacrosse days, Nate, just out of college, recalls the day when early in his study, full of skepticism, the class focused on a few individuals with persistent pain. The teacher prescribed a standing qigong for each individual and surrounded them with others doing particular movements as well.

> He had me standing doing standing Repulse Monkey—
> part of the meditation form that I've learned. And he put,
> I think four or six people stationed around me in a very
> particular placement relative to me. And they were all doing
> different parts of the form. He explained how one person
> is drawing energy in. Another person is drawing it up and
> [another] was sort of over here on my left behind me; he was
> supposed to be pulling something, like drawing out of me.

Discussing the exercise afterwards, Nate realized that what he felt was an absence of his ever present pain. He was able to walk and jump and was stunned to remain completely pain free for over a week.

Health changes are not just noticeable by those with obvious complaints. In her early twenties, Chenoa has become more conscious of what is going on in her body. She can feel the onset of a cold much earlier and often alter its course, lessening its severity or derailing it altogether through extra qigong and rest.

The key principles at play in manifesting changes in health, according to Roosevelt Gainey, who has guided a remarkable number of people through recovery from debilitating illnesses, are breathing and alignment.

61

The most important thing you have to do is breathe. You really can't breathe if you don't sit right. You can't meditate if you don't sit right. You fall in moving meditation if it's crunched up inside of you. Your skeleton has to be free to move. So if the skeleton supports the body, then the muscles move, energy will flow unimpeded and energy will go where it needs to fix you. I teach everybody—somebody with cancer the same thing as somebody with a cold. I teach you the same exact thing. It doesn't have to be a specific move to cure a specific thing. It's movement itself done correctly that will balance and bring the body back into oneness. When the body is in oneness, the natural internal healing mechanism kicks in.

Rosie's complete conviction comes from his personal experience after being near-fatally injured at a construction job.

I bled out. They told me I was going to have organ failure. And I found the same moves I was doing was giving me my strength back. They told me if I left the hospital, I was going to die. I signed myself out. And I started doing the simplest breathing, but in alignment. I couldn't walk from here to there [gestures]. It took me about 20 minutes.

I laid on my bed, and I did the breathing. It took me from morning to the afternoon to even go to the bathroom. Within a week I was able to walk to the boardwalk; the boardwalk is about two and a half blocks from my apartment. Once I got on the boardwalk, I'm doing my exercise, breathe, I walk from here to about there, sit down. Do some more. Walk. Sit. One day this lady in a wheelchair came by. A little old lady. She says, "What you doing?

I say "I'm trying to get my strength back." "Can I do it with you?" Six months later, we were power walking down the boardwalk.

Many miraculous stories revolve around taiji evangelists, but changes in outlook and health most often take place by degrees. This is due, in part, to a paradoxical phenomenon: many who have a glimpse of life without pain retreat in fear. Some [stories] says Laddie,

> ... are so profound as to almost appear phony. ... But when somebody is engaged with you in a series of exercises and suddenly shrieks in fear but then begins to cry and says "I'm not feeling the pain in my neck anymore," ... I guess a piece of intelligence that I've gained is that some people learn to strongly identify with their pain and can't give it up. And then if they accidently do have the experience without that pain, it's terrifying because its part of their personality that's being given up. If there's nothing to replace that void with, they're going to take the pain back.

Eli discovered taiji over thirty years ago, when he was a very young man. In his fifties, a mysterious lump on the side of his head was diagnosed as lymphoma. Remarking on the fact that Eli didn't look sick, his doctor encouraged him to continue with his taiji practice. Suffering from the side effects of chemo, that took some willpower, says Eli. "I'd walk outside and force myself to do the form to fight against it. I wouldn't let myself be sick. I used my energy, my internal energy to walk. ... Once I got into it, it was like nothing. I let it take over me."

Key, perhaps, to Eli's story was "getting into it." Eli does not just go through the motions of the form. He has a lifetime of disciplined and focused practice and an accepting nature of what is happening around him that allows him to move easily from the physical dimensions of the practice into the mind and spirit.

> I think it has a lot to do with breathing—connecting breathing to movement. I don't know if you ever did your form where it makes you moan?
> I think that's the connection right there. Connect everything with the circulation with your dantien. Everything is moving and all of a sudden go "mmmm." It goes through the whole body."

I experienced [the process of death] with the cancer. Everybody was telling me, "Eli, you handled this so well." You accept. I saw death is here. It's going to happen anyway. … What bothered me was the people that I loved and wanted to be around. So I didn't dwell on death; I just started living instead of thinking about dying.

Clearly Eli made the mind, body, spirit connections necessary to overcome such a serious illness. The psychological willingness to accept what was happening and to live the life he loved, for the people he loved, with the taiji practice that he loved, allowed a new balance to take hold. Over ten years later, he shows no signs of lymphoma and spends his retirement practicing daily as well as teaching boxing to neighborhood kids in his Brooklyn, New York garage.

Qi and Shifts in Consciousness

The mind, perhaps, is the hardest of the three elements to adjust, as evidenced by thousands of years of spiritual and philosophical writing examining its role and its illusions. However, the invitation to allow oneself to be psychologically flexible, creative, and imaginative is built into taiji through the Daoist use of metaphor, such as the five elements, animal frolics, golden pills, and names of the postures— Fair Lady Weaves the Shuttles, Golden Cock Stands on One Leg, or Old Man Plays Guitar.

The opposite can happen, too, if we react from fear and close ourselves to the possibilities that raised consciousness offers. People who are not willing to open to these possibilities quit pretty quickly. For those that stick it out, the opening and relaxing of the body begins to allow energy to flow through its meridians. Changes in mood or emotion are a part of the phenomenon, just as lowering stress and blood pressure might be.

David Hawkins' methodology describes negative thought patterns or attitudes that persist over time as being associated with an attractor energy field of corresponding power or weakness.

The result is a particular perception of the world, and appropriate events are created to trigger the specific emotion. All attitudes, thoughts, and beliefs are also connected with ... meridians of energy, to all of the body's organs. Through kinesiologic testing, it can be demonstrated that specific acupuncture points are linked with specific attitudes, and the meridian, in turn, serves as the energy channel to specific muscles and body organs" (Hawkins, 2002, p. 216).

Carole often finds that doing qigong or the form will lead to an emotional experience rather than a physical one.

[It] becomes a releasing experience. The other day we did some work touching the earth. We were sitting, and something was *really* touching my heart. What's interesting is to feel that energy touching my heart and whatever is caught in there. I cried a little bit because that was what needed to be released. But I also know not to contract around it. Just to open around that. To breathe into it.

Scientific research on taiji practitioners mostly addresses specific health benefits, such as its effects on arthritis or stress symptoms, as opposed to overall changes in consciousness. However, neuroscientists have done extensive mapping of brain functions of the phenomenon in yoga practitioners. Even though yoga trains you to concentrate on energy at the chakras while taiji trains energy to move through the meridians, many manifestations of qi may be equated with kundalini rising through the chakras. Each of the chakras also corresponds to a major point on those meridians (see Figure 1, page 71).

The biography of Master Kwan Saihung describes a chakra meditation that suggests that just as Daoism and Zen practices cross-fertilized, so have other meditation practices. Born in 1920 and sent to a Daoist monastery as a child, Saihung was of the last generation of taiji masters to be immersed in traditional Daoist training and education before the Japanese occupation of China. Similar to Indian kundalini meditation, the advanced *ling qiu* meditation he described opened the psychic centers sequentially from the base of the spine to the top of the crown to attain stillness and opening psychic powers.

The Grand Master continually warned Saihung that the abilities that would come to him would be gifts from the gods and were not to be abused. Many ascetics, having come this far, had fallen because they had grown obsessed with the importance of their centers. Instead of reaching the spiritual, they remained fascinated with the use of their lower centers and became trapped in the abuse of their powers.

Before he meditated to awaken each center, Saihung studied that center's colors and response to invocation, and looked at a diagram of its shape. Each center was imagined as a lotus bud that could be opened by the specific sound of the invocation. Within the flower was a certain pattern of colors. While he concentrated on that pattern in meditation, Saihung produced the invocation. The blooming center lit up, and its powers began to emanate. Saihung felt whirling sensations and heat whenever the center was activated. When the meditation was complete, the center closed and became dormant again.

… [H]e entered his final center. He was on the threshold of a level that was at once a culmination of many arduous years and the foundation for higher states; the Crown Center. The Thousand-Petaled Lotus bloomed. His senses dropped away. There was no external reality, no internal reality. He felt nothing, thought nothing. He merged completely with Voidness (Deng, 1993, pp. 120–2).

Brain researcher Erik Hoffmann and neurotherapist Inger Spindler describe a similar set of manifestations when kundalini awakens. Hearing sounds, seeing light, seeing the environment as illuminated, or other visual hallucinations are common. So is the feeling of unusual heat or cold as well as sensations of tickling, vibrating, itching, crawling—pleasant or unpleasant—within the body

66

or on the skin. Some experience kriyas—spontaneous, involuntary movements or positions of the body—in kundalini practice (Hoffmann, 2007) that are similar to many accounts from taiji players that we'll explore later.

Bruce Lipton's biological explanation is that cell membranes act as receptor "antennas" that:

> ... read vibrational energy fields such as light, sound and radio frequencies. The antennas on these "energy" receptors vibrate like tuning forks. If an energy vibration in the environment resonates with a receptor's antenna, it will alter the protein's charge, causing the receptor to change shape. ... Biological behavior can be controlled by invisible forces, including thought, as that provides the scientific underpinning for pharmaceutical-free energy medicine (Lipton, 2005, pp. 83–4).

Ma Jiannan, a professor of chemistry and director of the Engineering Institute at Hong Kong Chinese University makes the case that what we feel in our hands doing qigong is magnetic resonance. Our blood cells, which contain water and organic compounds, including iron, interact with the magnetic line force of the earth creating that feeling of a current (Ma, 1988).

In summary, sensations experienced by taiji practitioners are indicative of the interplay between qi and the body, as well as qi's ability to expand consciousness into the suprasensory dimensions. *The Secret of the Golden Flower* teaches us:

> What causes you to flow and revolve is just the six sense organs; but what enables you to attain enlightenment is also just the six sense organs. But the fact that sense objects and sense consciousnesses are not used at all does not mean using the sense organs; just using the essence in the sense organs (Cleary, 2000, p. 307).

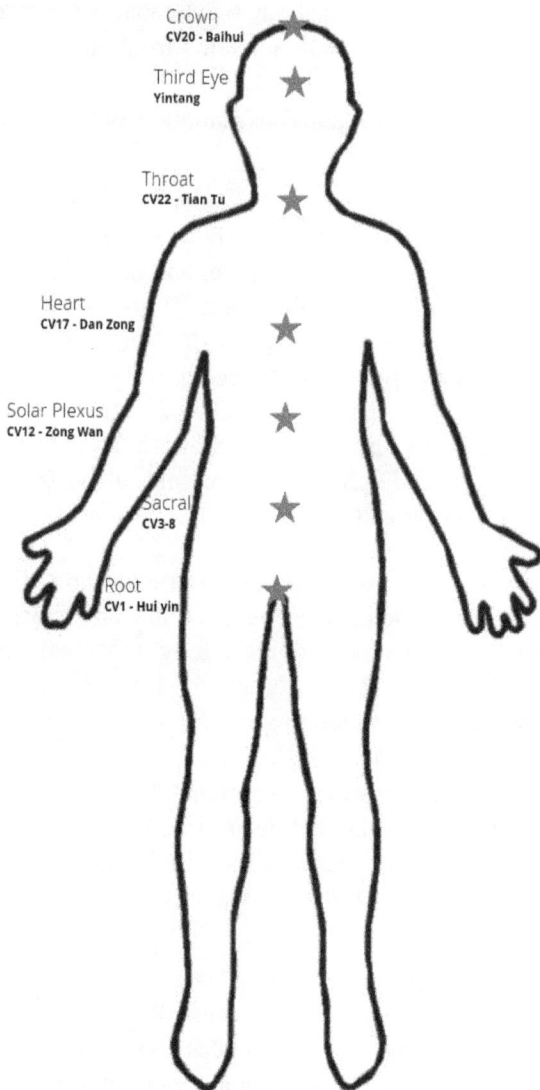

Crown
CV20 - Baihui

Third Eye
Yintang

Throat
CV22 - Tian Tu

Heart
CV17 - Dan Zong

Solar Plexus
CV12 - Zong Wan

Sacral
CV3-8

Root
CV1 - Hui yin

Figure 1

Accidents Avoided and Real Life Martial Situations

Tai chi chuan has no opinion. It has no intention. It is an idea without motive.

It is an act without desire. It is, properly, the natural response to an outside force, not being perceived as such.

For in nature, all are the same, everything is one. That which attacks is the same as that which responds, the same force – redirected and recycled.

When you initiate an ill-intentioned move, it comes back on you.

The principles of tai chi are the same principles behind the inner mechanism of the great engine of the universe.

—Cheng Man Ching (Cheng)

Heightened response to the potentially dangerous is another common phenomenon among taiji players. It is fair to say that avoiding an accident is really not substantially different from avoiding injury in a martial situation. Both can be seen as fear responses, and that is what we train for.

Video clips show Cheng Man Ching effortlessly sending opponents flying across a lawn and masters pushing a lineup of men like dominoes. These feed the imaginations of many a martial arts screenwriter. To do this requires deep development of *jing* (essence) through long and extensive standing practices. These standing *ichuan* practices develop both relaxed musculature and alignment to the earth's energy that facilitate a state of consciousness that allows one to transcend use of body strength, or *li* (Dong and Raffill, 2006, pp. 68–9).

On the receiving side, martial artists often take strenuous blows to their bodies in practice without having any damage done to them at all. Ken Van Sickle explains there are three ways you can take a strike to the body. "You can become tense, creating an ironlike stomach à la the legendary Harry Houdini. Second, you can fill with air pneumatically. This will allow you to take a blow, but risks damage to the kidneys. Third, you can relax. If you have any tension at all, it does not work—just like the rest of taiji." That deep cellular relaxation takes tremendous intention and hard work. Tension, even on a cellular level, can be broken.

> I remember the first time I saw that actually happen. Bruce Frantzis was a big powerful guy. At that time, he weighed about 250. His kick could kill you. He had a student who was about 5' 8" and weighed 135 pounds who, in front of a whole audience, took a full powered kick in the stomach. Then he came back and kicked him full power right in the solar plexus and knocked him down. But [the student] got up smiling.

The absorption of those deadly kicks was proof for Ken of the power of relaxation.

Eli's taiji has prevented injury several times. Twice in one week he was hit by a car while riding his racing bike as fast as he could on the streets of New York City. "I didn't get hurt; I just relaxed in the qi." After the second time though, he acknowledges he should have died and gave the racing bike away.

Bruce Walker also has seen the training as a literal lifesaver on more than one occasion. Once, when he was young and reckless, he fell off of the front of a Mercedes that was going at 30 miles an hour. He hit the ground, took two steps and fell. He instinctively rolled due to his martial arts training and came out with just a few scratches and scars.

Learning to fall into shoulder rolls is a routine part of all of Bruce's kung fu classes and many people told him how those lessons saved their lives.

> About ten years ago, a mother called me at two o'clock in the morning. Her child had been in my class, and he'd gone out riding with some friends and got into a really bad accident. Two of the kids were dead. One was in intensive care. He walked away, with minor scratches and she asked him "How did you live? How did you live when they died?" He replied, "I relaxed and rolled with it."

70

Maria noticed better balance and being more limber. Once she fell backward, tripping over a milk crate with her baby daughter on her arm. "It felt like slow motion," said Maria. She landed on the floor and picked herself up speaking in a reassuring voice. She did not drop the baby, nor did the baby make a peep. "That would not have happened if I hadn't been doing taiji."

Michelle remembers extensive work with peripheral vision in class, with exercises such as standing in the middle of a circle and having water bottles thrown at you while you tried to catch them. The results of that training revealed itself in the grocery store.

> I was [standing] there reading an egg carton to see whether it had the good omega-3s or the chickens were happier, or whatever. I'm just reading and paying no attention to anything else. An egg carton from a higher shelf fell down. Well, I just kept reading, caught the egg carton, and put it back. And I didn't even pay attention that I was doing it, and this guy next to me said "Nice catch, lady!"

Most of us are not presented with real life violent conflicts that truly test our accomplishments as martial artists. Some people would say that one measure of the success of training is they no longer find themselves in such situations, either because they are not seeking them out, they diffuse them before they become physical, or they have an air of confidence on the street that does not make them an inviting target. Some admit that their initial display of skill upon attack was enough to save them from nasty street fights.

Push hands training fosters listening, response, and neutralization. In real life situations, the master can meet the negative energy of a street fighter from a different plane, one not motivated by fear or the desire to win. Don Miller found that taiji enables one to round the corner or turn back before you drive "over the edge of the cliff in a yang versus yang situation."

A major test greeted Tom D. in the vestibule of his building one evening. Returning to his 14th Street, New York City walkup after work, his key was an inch from the lock to his apartment door when he heard the unmistakable scuffling and moaning sounds of a mugging downstairs. First his conscience kicked in. Should he ignore his neighbor and enter the safety of his own apartment or turn around in suit and tie to dive back down three flights of stairs to face combat? He had no idea whether he'd be facing a gun, a knife, or a gang of guys.

So I put my bag down, and going down the stairs I made a real racket. And I go, "Hey," on the way down. At one point, Professor [Cheng Man Ching] was asked about martial yells, like the kia ... and he made one at Shr Jung [the studio] that absolutely stopped everybody in the room. If you're relaxed, it's like opera. It has an intensity that it doesn't have if some guy screams like he's a chicken being choked. It really sends out your intention that you mean business.

The second time I yelled out, I actually dropped into my center and made that yell. ... And as I clear the last landing on the way down this flight of stairs, I see one of my neighbors, a particularly weeny guy, I mean nice enough, but stooped over in the corner sort of shaking and the front doors just swinging closed.

... What did I get from this? Well, first of all the kia thing; the fact that that second time, I was getting into the zone, because I knew when I turned that corner, I was going to have to get into it. I'd been doing aikido in those days. You make your move, or they'll kill you.

... I understood that I was going into a moment that was going to be life altering for somebody. And that's what I meant about this isn't a game. We're not just playing around. I see guys pushing hands and doing stuff that, from a technical point of view, if you've done any other martial arts, you'll see that's a broken arm, that's a broken knee, that's a broken neck. Without qi, it's just leverage, nothing fancy. When we practice push hands it's point blank range because that's the moment of truth. The moment of actual contact. The rest is just dancing around making faces at each other.

... What counts is when you come into contact. Taiji

strips away everything. It's about spirit and contact. And you have to be deadly serious when your bodies are belly to belly because the slightest mistake in that range—that's the dead zone.

Exploding Objects and the Extraordinary

If you wish to upset the law that all crows are black, you mustn't seek to show that no crows are; it is enough if you prove one single crow to be white.

—William James (James, 1897, p. 5)

There was a period of time a couple years into my practice, when I could feel myself opening more and more to qi. This corresponded with the lightest touch breaking wine glasses, favorite ceramic mugs, and a couple of teapots. Fortunately, that phase passed before the cupboards were bare. Around that time, we went to a memorial and luncheon for the wife of a taiji friend who had been studying for around 25 years. When he picked up my ceramic serving bowl to take to the kitchen for washing, it shattered. That synchronicity led me to the realization that such breakage was a result either of incoherent energy or an uncontrolled or unintended *fa jin*, an explosive discharge of energy, like a sneeze. Our friend, although a very advanced player, broke the bowl on a day when he was under extreme emotional strain, however composed he outwardly appeared. As I advanced in my study, this phenomenon passed, as it did for many of the students from a school nearby.

David Chandler, as you may recall, experienced an exploding milk bottle early on in his practice. That lightest touch triggered great drama, but through further awareness and study, energy seemed to settle into other patterns for him.

Lynn was among David's students when a number of people from the school also had glass shattering experiences. The group, many of whom had been practicing for several years, had been practicing bone breathing and exercises where you move to the left when you think to the right. One person put his hand through a car window. Not realizing the window was there, he simply put his hand through the clear glass—shattering it, but not hurting himself. Lynn set a ceramic drinking cup down by the sink. She noted that it made an unusually sharp and snappy sound. Then as she brushed her teeth, she tried to scrape off a hair with her finger and discovered a crack in the solid white porcelain pedestal.

Shortly thereafter, she took a cereal bowl out of the cabinet and it, too, exploded in her hand. "It was like something just went through me. I was totally open and not in my body. I channeled whatever the energy was to make the dish explode."

Another night in class, the group practiced punching into a partner's open palm. After some extended practice something clicked for Lynn. She asked her partner to let her try once more.

> He put out his hand, and I felt it come up through my leg. It was perfectly lined up and I felt it just go through me. I punched him and it just was just like putting that cup down on the sink. This look went over his face, and it kind of vibrated his whole body. This was a guy who had boxed in the army. He looked at me and started laughing. His shoulder and back hurt for a couple hours afterwards. I didn't feel the impact on his hand; it felt like I had done nothing.

In Rick K.'s story, the drinking glass started sliding away from him and exploded as as his hand got within an inch or two of it as his son sat watching. At this point Rick had felt qi flowing into him during push hands, but had not felt the sensation of qi running through him. Then one day, he shattered the glass shower door. "I was about to touch it, and it just completely exploded." He, too, felt nothing when the glass shattered.

Bruce Lipton explains the phenomenon:

When, for example, a skilled vocalist like Ella Fitzgerald maintains a note that is harmonically resonant with the atoms of a crystal goblet, the goblet's atoms absorb her sound waves. Through the mechanics of constructive interference, the added energy of resonant sound waves causes the goblet's atoms to vibrate faster. Eventually the atoms absorb so much energy that they vibrate fast enough to break free from the bonds that hold them together. When that happens, the goblet actually explodes (Lipton, 2005, p. 118).

A teacher's influence in the experience of qi, conscious or not, is real. Maggie Newman leads the form with the intent to create unity within the room as well as with the ground, body, heaven, earth, and you in between:

The experience is nonseparateness. That feels good. It makes the experience feel comfortable. … if I can be with the group, as in my movement, then I get the advantage of not just my qi, but the group qi. Which is like a huge person doing taiji. I get the value of that, and the pleasure of that, and the nonseparateness of that. I think the experience of nonseparateness is joy and happiness. And the experience of separateness is pain, loneliness, sadness, and isolation. … I enjoy experiences of the oneness with people through movement.

Through entrainment, energetic coherence can grow within a group. It would make sense for that to be the case in all schools, intentionally or not. That is not to say that any teacher sets out to have their students breaking glass doors and dishes, but, when individuals and groups open and allow themselves to surrender, things start to happen. As David Chandler sees it,

There are patterns. There are cycles. Sometimes cycles in a group—who comes to taiji class, for instance. There are patterns in individuals as well, and, yet, every person is unique. And that's one of the things that taiji does, I think. It helps each individual unfold into his individuality.

Even though we're all doing the same move, it's going to be done slightly differently because their tensions are in different places. ... I can see generally, "Ok this is where you're coming from. You are in a lot of pain, physical pain, emotional pain. You have some arrogance." You see these things, and you see that they're going to get polished. So they come in kind of rough. Sometimes with a rough edge and even sometimes scowls on their faces, like prove to me that what you're doing is good for me. "You know, I've heard all this stuff, and I just don't believe it." Some of the toughest people will have the largest transformations.

The implication that something greater is going on can also be more direct. One day, Bob stood at the back of a line of people pushing against the teacher. The teacher suddenly turned that force around. Everybody in that line felt something, but only Bob, at the back of the line, got thrown.

Chris, ever the skeptic, did a public demonstration with Stephe one day. Standing twenty feet behind Chris, Stephe directed his intent without any touching, and moved him from side to side.

That's got to be really hard to do. It's got to be harder to do to someone who doesn't believe it can be done, and he did it to me repeatedly. He figured out which way he was going to push me, and that's the way I went. I have absolutely no explanation for it except that when something happens to you, you pretty much have to accept that it happened to you.

Perhaps, because such stories are the stuff of legends, Newtonian thinkers are quick to dismiss them and dismiss all live or video evidence of the mysterious as undetected fraud. Like William James' white crow, however, there are so many firsthand accounts like Chris' and Bob's, as well as of modern masters like Cheng Man Ching and T.T. Liang, that it is impossible to rationally dismiss the body of experience without revealing an entrenched bias.

What sets these masters apart so that they achieve at such a consistently authentic level? Cheng Man Ching told his students, the difference between them was they only practiced taiji in class, but he did taiji all the time. Whether his taiji took the form of healing, calligraphy, painting, poetry, eating, walking, or socializing, he operated from a state of completely integrated body, mind, spirit.

Rick Barrett points to Yang Fukui, as a living master who lives and teaches in New York City. Fukui is particularly adept at isolating the qualities of the five elements—wood, fire, earth, metal, or water—so that they are distinct. The five elements in taiji or Chinese healing are a coherent whole, much like white light is an assimilation of the entire color spectrum, or how timbre in sound is derived from the relative strength of overtones. "They're all part of one fundamental energy. In healing what you're doing is feeling into where the deficiency is. Where is the excess?" The healer can then either promote the missing element or remove excess to promote balance.

Don Miller, reflecting on some of his extraordinary experiences, realizes that they maybe were not quite as extraordinary as he once believed.

I think, to some degree, it is replicable if I go back and think about what I was doing. Maybe it was the Irish whiskey, but it's also a certain thought process that produces a physiological and/or energetic change that can be quite profound. And, in fact, a lot of my taiji discoveries of the last 10 years have been realizing that there are hundreds of these little switches or triggers, some of which are just thoughts or specific kinds of instructions you give yourself that produce instantaneous alteration in your state with far greater objective results than you could possibly imagine. I mean people do one exercise and it seems like they got 10 years of taiji better. So a lot of my work these days is just experimenting and cataloguing a lot of those triggers and switches and processes that jump you into some other state.

Recalling that Cheng Man Ching said, "It's not magic, it's real," Don agrees.

Taiji does have within its array of offerings, some really amazing stuff that on the surface might seem magical, but as you put your decades into it, you realize it's not magic, it's real. It's just stuff that you get to by building up a succession of other skills. And it doesn't end.

Becoming Healers

[A]ll things that have consciousness depend upon breath. But if they do not get their fill of breath, it is not the fault of Heaven. Heaven opens up the passages and supplies them day and night without stop. But man on the contrary blocks up the holes. The cavity of the body is a many-storied vault; the mind has its Heavenly wanderings. But if the chambers are not large and roomy, then the wife and mother-in-law will fall to quarreling. If the mind does not have its Heavenly wanderings, then the six apertures of sensation will defeat each other.

—Zhuangzi (Watson, 2003, p. 35)

It is a common rite of passage for taiji players to open up to their own healing abilities. Qi, interpreted through different lenses, can be manipulated on a martial level, a healing level, or in joint endeavors such as chamber music or team sports. Depending on our intent, we can sense the energy of another person and push it away, neutralize it, merge with it, or facilitate a harmonious healing vibration. Common to all three is the 'listening' aspect, whereby one takes in information on suprasensory levels and acts on that information. In the Daoist healing traditions, this listening is first encountered with the reading of the pulses. Then, with herbs, acupuncture, *tui na* (a form of massage or body work informed by meridian theory), or medical qigong, one proceeds to regain balance in the meridians, either by slowing down a stream, opening a blockage, or stimulating a sluggish flow. With better balance, comes ease (as opposed to dis-ease) and better health. The principles are in play in less circumscribed healing arts as well, such as reiki and distance healing.

Residing in that blurred boundary where the ethereal plane and physical plane intersect, remote healers such as Shirdi Sai Baba or Edward Cayce demonstrated the quantum nature of our bodies in space. To affect a change in an individual from afar using intent and mental concentration depends on a unified field of consciousness. There, one can tap into the "self-generating feedback loop across the cosmos" (McTaggart, 2008, p. 20). That ability allowed Edward Cayce to provide insight and diagnosis in a trance state to thousands of people, with an estimated 85 percent accuracy. Likewise, both Shirdi Sai Baba and Sathya Sai Baba produced well documented and miraculous results for disciples around the world as well as in their local ashrams.

Scholars, including William James, have studied psychic phenomena for generations. Investigations of distance healing through intent have shown measurable effects on cells, water, animals, and plants (Schwartz, 2017). Yet, in the realm of clinical trials, materialistic methods have only showed minor effect, largely due to poor study design using methods ill-suited to the phenomenon (Radin et al., 2015). Just one experience in this realm though can change one's mind about healing methods that go back thousands of years and across cultures.

One beautiful autumn day driving to the Berkshires on business, a call arrived from the school bus ferrying my ten-year-old son and his classmates to Boston from Connecticut for a field trip. He had mysteriously broken out in hives. He'd never had hives, so I attributed it to his over excitement. Not being the driver, I was able to concentrate on him to help clear his energy field. The school held off on giving him Benadryl and in a short while he was remarkably better. Had we been "separate" entities I doubt any energy could penetrate 100 miles, the steel of a car and school bus, and our separate bodies. But accepting the nondual, it makes sense that an open channel can be tuned into and helpful energy transmitted between people, even between people in two moving vehicles a hundred miles apart.

A Pentecostal, Bruce felt that his studies of martial arts helped him open the pathway to communication with spirits, and his faith in this was reinforced by his emerging healing ability.

> What really convinced me that I wasn't just BSing myself was when my wife started tattooing. I would go into her shop and start talking. A lot of times she would be working on somebody and that person was facing away from me. Generally, I'd just nod to her, and start talking with her boss. If she had somebody there in a lot of pain, I started doing spiritual healing. And every time I tried it, after two or three minutes, the guy would start to relax, to breathe. Instead of having tense shoulders, his shoulders would go down. His body would drop like he wasn't hurting anymore. … That kind of convinced me I could produce some things.

Such ability to heal requires sensitivity and an ability to listen to qi and the information that arrives on nonrational levels. "The main sensory extraction that I experience is more like a kinesthetic knowledge. So it's more of a gut knowingness," says Leyla. "I can look at somebody; I can feel somebody—feel into them, but it's nonverbal."

Laddie also attunes to people on the psychic level:

> Sometimes I feel the typical trembly, tingly feeling. Sometimes I feel heat. Sometimes I feel a movement between me and the person I'm working on, but most of the time it's just a sense of knowing. You know when it's there, and you know when it's not.
>
> I don't see auras; I don't see colors; I don't see wave patterns. I just have a whole body experience of awareness.
>
> … When working with people directly and specifically for healing, I am immediately attuned to their emotional being. It's not a matter of I could tell you what the source

of the problem is, but I can tell you where the pain is being held, and feel that pain and be affected by it.

Asked to elaborate on the energetic distinctions between playing taiji and doing healing work, polarity therapist and taiji teacher Rick Barrett explains that the qualitative differences in energies between healing, meditative practice, and taiji martial practice center around intent.

Whenever I'm doing energy healing I'm looking for a compassionate neutrality. I'm seeking to find the centered place [in myself] to allow the energy to pivot around that.

It creates a relationship that, by going to the center, allows everything else to become exposed. And the body mind can then say "Oh, I don't need that particular energy pattern now. What am I hanging onto that for?" And it can let go. Sometimes you want to provoke a certain response because things are stuck and then you'll go for a specific quality of energy just to prime the pump. But as soon as you get it going, then you want to go back to that compassionate neutrality and allow it to unfold. For example, if someone is really stuck or indecisive you may want to provoke a fiery response by touching certain parts of the body or—what polarity's all about—a jausic touch—a gentle rocking will produce a fiery response. That will get things going. Once things are going, then you can allow that to unfold.

Whereas in taiji, you're definitely working with the energies, and you're more consciously directing the flow of the energies and how they are expressed. If I'm doing a meditative form, the quality of my energy may be watery. I just kind of want to get in the flow and just let the form kind of flow. But, I may be seeking a more martial aspect. I may want a fiery quality to it or a metal quality to it, something that would be good for more of a martial situation. And to really get the taiji, you have to do the whole palette and all combinations in between.

Shake, Rattle, and Roll—The Weird, Wondrous, and Wonted

One mind produces the right concentration,
Myriad forms are spontaneously arrayed,
Five energies are distributed through the quarters.
The five energies are pregnant with one spirit,
The one spirit pervades transformation,
Crystallizing and refining the original reality.
The original reality is not something with form:
It is neither existent nor nonexistent.
If people can penetrate this principle,
Then they'll understand the pearl that unifies sense experience.

—Sun Bu-er (Cleary, 2000, pp. 434–5)

Proprioception, one's perception of stimuli and the feelings inside one's own body, is an area that many taiji teachers choose not to discuss. Some feel that it interferes with the practice by setting up an expectation or desire based on someone else's experience. On the other hand, beginners sometimes think there is something abnormal about their sensations or that maybe they are doing something wrong if they feel something different from others in their cohort. Lack of discussion does not serve them well, whereas open mindedness is a neutral platform from which to allow one's own development to transpire, especially in a culture where mystical experiences and body mind practices are on the cultural fringe. In fact, the drama of physical manifestations is key for many people beginning their studies. It is an affirmation that there is something to the practice and a point of entry to deeper understanding of the Dao. If a backdrop of no expectation is firmly in place, bodily perceptions offer a safe topic of discussion among colleagues not accustomed to baring themselves to the greater conversations that mind and spiritual openings will require.

Modern teachers tend to focus their classes on body mechanics, health, and to a lesser extent the martial art. Even the Chinese masters

Da Liu and B.P. Chan, who taught in New York City beginning in the 70s, leaned toward the form, push hands, and meditation techniques rather than spiritual aspects, said Reggie Jackson.

> [They taught] everything through feeling not through thinking. … Feeling the energy around you, feeling through push hands, where the touch of the hands tells you where it is. … and even feeling when you're not touching hands.

The fact is, spiritual discovery and mystical experience do arise through taiji practice. For those with overactive minds, approaching the practice proprioceptively can move one away from an entrenched sense of self and will and will shift into the witness level of consciousness, especially if one does not immediately start creating narratives to explain such manifestations of qi. Those who overemphasize the physical body risk missing out on nondual discovery by being stuck on the physical level (Liao, 2010, pp. 64–6).

Even those whose initial focus is on health delve deeper than just feeling one's most obvious physical and emotional aches and pains dissolve. Roosevelt Gainey, whose teaching revolved around the breath and proper function, or alignment, recalled a taiji player with 30 years of experience who came to him after being diagnosed with cancer. Despite those 30 years it was the first time he really felt qi. Questioning *what* he was feeling and *where* in his body he was feeling it, Rosie explained to him that, "Whatever your body's doing, you're supposed to be doing. Your body has an innate wisdom. When you give it the proper things it needs, it will take care of itself. You don't have to do anything."

Typical of beginning students, Tom D. didn't feel qi during his first three years of practice, even though it was a source of great conversation, idle speculation, and doubt.

> You wonder, is it qi? Is it just a pinched nerve? Is it real? Then, it was as if I was blinking my eyes and waking up in the morning. I'd have a moment where I'd sort of feel something that wasn't the same as just grinding my way

physically through the form. And then I'd try to capture it, and it would of course elude me. I guess the best way to describe it is that after about three years I started to more consistently feel myself in a different space—in a zone where it sort of felt a little warm. If I was in a certain position relative to myself, and all the parts of my body got into a certain kind of alignment, it would be there. If I was just a little out of line, it would be gone.

Or as Nina remembers with wide, wondrous eyes, years later, "It was like a miracle to know that I have it."

Linda, a computer programmer by day, poet and fiction writer by night, describes feeling like a cellphone on vibrate, down to the bone level, and feeling a shudder going through her body. When she's able to let herself become part of everything around her she has moments when she recognizes herself physically as just being a waveform. Those moments are characterized by a general sense of lightness in which she could actually defy gravity by floating away. "It just comes out," she says, "somewhat like laughter."

Eli, like many taiji players, supplements his studies with yoga. Yoga's different physical approach of moving energy through chakras rather than meridians unlocks physical tightness and loosens the joints in a different way than taiji does. Going into the corpse position one day led Eli to an unmistakable experience of qi in which he felt himself let everything go—his whole body and spirit. "It was like I wasn't there. When I came back I was like I'd been asleep. Where did I go? It was scary at first."

Now, practicing in a much softer manner than he had for many years, Eli feels a lot of qi. His experience is that if your movements are soft you feel it open your body and that on occasion leads to spontaneous moaning. "Moaning only comes when you're totally soft, and your breathing is connected with the movement."

Bruce described heightened awareness to his senses taking in the world around him, but also his internal landscape.

84

I'm more aware of everything around me. Not that my hearing is more acute or my sense of smell is more acute, but I'm mindful of what my senses mean. I see something out of the corner of my eye; I tend to look at it. I tend to be aware of that. If I smell something funny, I hear something funny, I turn around very quickly.

... But also, it feels like my body's humming, but my body's not really humming. It kind of feels like my body did when I took acid or drugs, but its not like who I felt like when I took acid. I can feel my body working, I guess. That's difficult to put into words—but I go through my life feeling like I'm really connected in some ways to a lot of things. And in some ways, connected to everything.

Leyla's early experiences were typical with the sensations of buzzing, tingling, and generally feeling a lot better than usual. It was the first time that she really started feeling her body and what it felt like to move the arm on a minute level.

Similarly, Chenoa describes a warm fuzzy happy feeling in her hands and feet. That developed into strongly feeling the point in the middle of her palms and the sensation that her arms were resting on air instead of her muscles holding them.

Inez observes that her bodily experience varies tremendously from day to day. "One of the main signs I've had that the qi is really being more supportive as I do the form is in the amount of relaxation I'm able to incur in my upper body."

Sensations in the hands are the most commonly talked about, perhaps because we use our hands as our primary touch sensors. Eli recalls driving his teacher, Ming, home from practice in a Brooklyn park one day. Nearly an hour after they'd stopped working out, he still had bright red circles on the palms of his hands.

Gina found the sensations of qi peaceful with little "beats" massaging her body. She could also feel pressure between the hands or the feeling of air in the spaces between her hands. Sometimes she also felt heat, but more interesting to her was what it revealed.

It was profound. You can actually sense not only our body and space, but the other bodies in spaces as they're doing their work. It reminded me a lot of what a great ballet class was, in terms of doing exercises together to the rhythm of music. This was without music, but the music was there in the air, in the flow of the movements.

The body can also yield results that are both substantially and insubstantially dramatic. Through acupuncture, Christine had her first experience with qi. Feeling heat pour from the chest and circulate down her body, she was wowed. "This is what I've been missing all these years." A layer of fatigue lifted and she felt "150 percent awake," a state that lasted for four days.

Studying form, her day-to-day sensations vary from profoundly feeling "a lot" to sometimes not feeling anything at all. Christine describes openness as well as the weight in her body feeling in sync. She feels currents move through her body and the sense of weight in her hands, her hands connecting to her feet, her head connecting to her feet, and heat in the belly. The intensity varies with the quality of motion and lessens with quantity of motion.

A critically acclaimed modern dancer and teacher, Christine differentiates the experience of taiji from dance, which she equates with the feeling of being a bird in flight. In the Cheng Man Ching videos, she points out that Maggie Newman, also a professional dancer in her early decades, was so light. Forty years later her taiji revealed a deep saturation.

Tom M. also describes energy coming up through his feet and legs and through his arms. He feels his arm being lifted by the energy rather than it being a muscular action. At times the feeling of the connection between the full arm and full leg is apparent. "I can feel the difference between what that feels like and the cross connection between the empty leg and the empty arm. And then when I go to change, I feel the energy changing."

After time, extraordinary sensations seem ordinary. "Things happen every day, but what makes them interesting is their insubstantiality, which makes them less of a bar story and more of a meditation," says Rick Barrett who explains that any skill, even the ability to place attention on dissolving root in push hands, can become commonplace. Then every once in a while, circumstances such as a life or death situation, bring it back from the ordinary.

You start noticing what's not there. So if you use the idea of air—air is very insubstantial by comparison to this table, but when it starts to move around, you start to feel the sensations. "Oh, something's moving." … Or you'll notice "The air feels wet today. It's very moist." Consequently, you'll be able to perceive at a sensory level what's going on there. But after a while, you notice air for its insubstantiality as well—as a space holder. It is like noticing the space between thought becomes a very distinct thing. First you just notice the thoughts, then you start focusing on the space between. That is not unlike in music. You hear the notes; that's all you hear at first. And then, as you develop your ear, the pauses, the silences between the notes, are as eloquent as the notes themselves.

Moving deeper into the experience, Maria equates the sensation of qi with receiving.

It's like an extended touch. And in my body, I can feel a flow—an electrical, or tingling, or sometimes it's a glowing feeling. It's just a sensation of direction. It's like edges. Once you really get the qi going, the energy is not so much of an edge but a transition point.

In Maggie Newman's class, where there is a focus on the energy of the group, Tom M. is sometimes able to really tune into the other people in the room. He describes an arch of energy connecting the tops of everyone's heads and being shared by all.

Maybe it's just like the energy is there, like a quantum physics principle where, you know, you ask for the energy, and it's here. But I tend to visualize it as coming through me in an arch or rainbow … I perceive it as being colorful. I perceive it as it being more or less invisible, but palpable.

Maggie Newman first feels the substantiality of tension blocking the qi. Then, when feeling openness without any clenching or clutching, the entire body functions towards one end. She describes a warm wave of energy passing through the body into the ground.

If it's a good day, with no obstructions, it is as if I'm one with ground, and one with air, and one with heaven. I'm a channel that energy is flowing through into the ground and filling up. That feels luscious, and that makes me feel so grateful to be alive.

Many of the physical phenomena that people experience are simply releases of old or stagnant energy facilitated by the flow of qi. In my first year of taiji classes, every Saturday morning upon finishing the form, three people would head for the box of tissues, and the teacher would belch repeatedly. As Maria puts it, "If you're constipated you're going to fart a lot. If you've got a cold, your nose is going to be dripping." Maggie Newman has seen a lot of crying among beginning students as their bodies release long held or unresolved emotional issues:

Sometimes taiji is like water rolling over a rock and when that happens, the body may open up. Or there's a crystalized thing in the body, and that lock relaxes and carries with it an emotion.

Reggie Jackson laughed about classes with Master Da Liu because about three quarters of the way through the form, everyone started burping. "Da Liu always said it was getting rid of toxins. ... It was a remarkable thing that practically everyone we taught it to, had the same results." Da Liu was very concerned with being able to get a flow going through a state of relaxation. In *T'ai Chi Ch'uan and Meditation* he explains that belching and passing gas are common responses that can be refined over time.

When they happen and when they do not, both situations are good. The stomach and the intestines are "involuntary" organs: no amount of physical exercise alone can force them to move. But when the movements of T'ai Chi Ch'uan are performed correctly and the ch'i is directed by the mind to the abdomen, these organs may expand and constrict. Inhaling fresh air and exhaling the stale, you send cleansing blood and vitality to the vibrating organs. As a result, the digestion of food and the formation of wastes are expedited. Like the fumes from an automobile engine, gas is the byproduct of the digestive process. Since burping and flatulence are means by which the body eliminates impurities, they are healthy and good, although not graceful when done in public.

A more advanced stage occurs when the movements are performed more skillfully and are more coordinated with the mind and breathing in the abdomen. Use the mind to sink the chi down into the dantien to avoid burping. Then use your mind to constrict the anal sphincter so that the passageway becomes closed, forestalling the escape of gas. The air can then be kept inside the body as a form of energy. This means that you have attained the meditative phenomenon. (Liu, 1986, pp. 158–9)

Shaking is a less common but quite potent manifestation of qi as well. Bob, after shaking for several years in his practice, suddenly stopped when he switched teachers and learned a different qigong set.

For me, shaking developed gradually through standing practice. Over the course of a couple of years it felt like popcorn was erupting inside of me until one day, it broke outside of the body, and I became a full-throttled gyrating mass until my feet couldn't hold onto the ground. Explanations from teachers ranged from "it is incoherent energy," "kundalini rising," to sheer bafflement.

Reggie Jackson said that master BK Chan was very big on standing and also saw shaking as a release:

[Standing] opens the 13 joints—2 shoulders, 2 elbows, 2 wrists, 6 right? 2 knees, 2 ankles, right? 2 hips, right? And the spine counts as 1. That's 13. He [Chan] says, "Standing, relax. Just add a little bit every day. Don't try to do a half hour. " Chan, he stands an hour no problem. ... and some of these guys would be shaking. I said, "Chan, look, he's really shaking isn't he?" "Yea," he says, "even if I kill him, I make him healthy!"

Chan explained that shaking is evidence of the thirteen channels opening. When you get to the point that all thirteen channels open up, then everything will flow freely.

Moving deeper, Bradford Keeney's study of shaking through spiritual practices around the world led him to the conclusion that it is possible to get to deeper levels not only through meditation, but also through arousal:

> [W]e can sometimes get to the highest states of ecstasy through the opposite pathway—via meditative stillness and quiet. Ecstatic and meditative experiences are not separate. The co-presence of arousal and relaxation must be acknowledged when we speak of the self-regulating healing processes of the human body, mind, and soul (Keeney, 2007, p. 28).

Likewise, the medieval Jewish mystic Abulafia claimed fear and trembling a natural and essential part of the ecstatic process in which fear gives way to sensing spirit in the body (*Sitrei Torah*, Paris Ms. 774, fol. 158a). His guides to achieving prophetic experiences also included breathing exercises, body movements, and recitation of divine names and symbols.

> [A]nd your limbs begin to shake, and you will fear a tremendous fear [...] and the body will tremble, like the rider who races the horse, who is glad and joyful, while the horse trembles beneath him (*Otzar Eden Ganuz*, Oxford Ms. 1580, fols. 163b-164a; see also *Hayei Haolam Haba*, Oxford 1582, fol. 12a) (*Wikipedia*, 2016).

On the spiritual plane, a fundamentalist minister basking in the aftermath of a taiji form said, "It feels like forgiveness." That description is not dissimilar to crying as an emotional release. A sense of self, rigid perhaps in its righteousness, gives way to something softer. It is physically recognizable as an absence of substantiality. Forgiveness, like anger and joy, has a recognizable set of bodily characteristics—perhaps an easing of tension around the heart and neck, and the feeling of radiant light shining from within. Stepping away from the mind long enough to let the body become the focus of attention creates space from which such a change can sprout. Or, as Laddie interprets his student's experience, "Forgiveness probably needs to come from the self first. ... It's not fighting that wave."

At the conclusion of an intense and prolonged period of meditative movement, another of Laddie's students—a Catholic priest—said, "I feel like I'm in the state of grace that comes immediately after confession." Laddie points out that this greater experience of the student's culture is facilitated by an open mind:

> [I]f they're having a spiritual hunger or conflict, then their awareness of that may become heightened as a result of the practice. From a purely secular, physical human point of view, if you have some emotions that are stuck, that you've really been wrestling with, you might find yourself crying, or laughing, and not even know exactly why. You can give permission for that to happen, and it happens.

Even early in her study, Lynn found taiji had profound effects. She describes a "crawly ants in my arms kind of a feeling," as well as gradually becoming more balanced and peaceful, despite her first teacher's rather military approach to moving through forms. Describing a set of qigong exercise just a few months into her study, Lynn recalls:

> At the end I was standing there, and I just started to drool, sort of uncontrollably drooling. After class I asked her about it because it was just so weird. ... She got all excited, and said it was the **golden elixir** and that it was a really good thing and just keep following it.

Lynn is particularly sensitive on the physical level and shows ease in learning new moves and exercises. In addition to the extreme sensations of hot and cold in her fingers, she has also found them dripping. This phenomenon was most dramatic during a Tai Chi Alchemy workshop held in Sedona when the instruction was to lead the form with the hands, instead of having the expression come out of your hands. "I realized my fingers were dripping onto the floor. Nowhere else was I sweating. And it didn't even feel like sweat. It was just like water running."

Another time, when a class was doing the swimming dragon qigong, Lynn was really into the nuances of the s-curves and the transitions from crouching to standing. At the end, she found her hands wet, but rather than looking like sweat, the moisture was milky and translucent.

Chris Chorney has learned to go meditate when he is in the "worst mood possible." Even though he doesn't usually stand more than five or ten minutes he usually becomes soaked in perspiration, a phenomenon that does not extend to his form practice.

> I will sweat like I'm running a marathon and my feet will get really hot. After I'm done my palms will be very hot. I sit still and watch TV all the time and I don't get hot. I go ahead and I do a meditation where I'm doing less than I'm doing when I'm watching TV, and I generate all this heat.

And rather than being exhausted from an activity that engenders extreme perspiration, Chris finds he is energized by it.

Bob Messinger's experience is more aligned with descriptions in the Chinese classics than most people report. Physically, he sensed qi through the bottom of the feet and at the top of the head at the bai hui point.

> [I]t's in perfect balance in the middle when the connection is made. The body becomes firm but balanced and at the same time relaxed and soft. And the mind becomes quiet and soft. It's much like what I've had all my adult life, growing up with my connection to nature. It's that same kind of feeling of wonder and awe, but at the same time [has] confidence and power.

Entering the Mystical Zone

The Universal Energy Dance

> *It is said that we are the same in essence but different in feeling. There is no difference in feeling either; it is just that habits develop unnoticed, evolving in a stream, continuing to the present, so that their defiling influence cannot be shed. Ultimately this is not the fault of essence.*

—The Secret of the Golden Flower (Cleary, 2000, p. 320)

Cloaked in the vessel of the body and the garments of mind it is easy to obscure the fundamental premise of nonduality—that we are Dao. In recent years, through quantum physics, and its application to biology and biochemistry, science has begun to align itself behind this prime reality.

Physicists have taught us that all matter is composed of energy, coagulated energy that takes the dual forms of particles and waves. From that point of view, the difference between the energy of a thought and my bones becomes a difference in frequency. Energetic waves can change frequency, merge with other waves, or decay. When two waves merge they may harmonize, gain resonance, and flow more freely.

Taiji promotes shifts in body mechanics that allow the life force energy emanating from Dao, qi, to gradually soften habits creating internal tension and blockages, or to release held energetic patterns, thus promoting healing and a sense of wholeness through its circulation. When rooted and aligned in the structure of the body, taiji players are able to tap into the energy of the earth and the surrounding air, allowing change in one's relationship with one's own *jing* (inner essence). That results in vibration with greater coherence and amplitude in relation to external forces and, perhaps, inner calm.

Music as a Metaphor

Music and musical instruments offer a useful metaphor for understanding this paradox. All sound is generated by vibration, and pitch is determined by a fundamental or root frequency. Musical tone is shaped by overtones, neatly mapped out by Pythagoras, that are responsible for the color and quality of musical sound. The first overtones are the consonants: the octave, then a perfect fifth and a perfect fourth above that. Then shades of the imperfect consonants enter the spectrum, through the thirds and sixths. Lastly we reach the dissonant sevens, seconds, and tritone. This pattern continues well beyond the frequencies audible by the human ear.

Now imagine that you and I are different instruments in the orchestra. We can each play a beautiful A, but they will not sound the same. The A of an oboe is not the same as the A of the violin or trumpet, despite sharing the same fundamental pitch. That difference in sound quality is timbre. Timbre is the spectral compilation of a fundamental and its overtones. The bell tones of the brass family have strong octaves, fifths, and fourths. The rich moodiness of the oboe is colored by the relative strength of the thirds and sixths. The determinants of those overtones are the shape of the resonating body, the materials it is made from, and its means of creating the vibration, i.e., buzzing air through a metal mouthpiece, blowing through two slices of reed cane, pulling a bow across a string, plucking a string, etc.

When combined, tones of two instruments played by competent musicians tune to each other, gaining harmonic resonance. This "intensification and enriching of a musical tone by supplementary vibration" (Webster, 2016) may emanate from the air surrounding an oscillating string or the bell of a wind instrument. Or it may come from another instrument or player of the same instrument. When you hear an exquisitely tuned ensemble, you will notice how rich, juicy, and alive the sound is. The blended sound, tuned perfectly, shimmers and can sometimes even amplify difference tones (extremely high pitches created by the combined overtones to create a phantom voice in the aural harmony).

Now think of our bodies as instruments. Some are tall and skinny; some are short and plump. Some are toned; some are soft. Some are sinewy; some are lithe. Some are diseased; some are stressed. Some are young and resilient; some are leathered by sun and age. These vessels of infinite individuality are resonators, just like the wooden body of the acoustic guitar or the curvaceous brass bell of the saxophone. Individuality can be seen as a byproduct of the resonating chambers that shape the quality of your voice, the quality of your emotions, and the color of your aura. In other words, your personality, habits, quirks, and emotions are reflected, or amplified, in your spectral output.

Let's assume that the root frequency for everyone is determined by the earth's qi. It is transmitted through the ground at what is known as the Schumann resonance, or approximately at 7.8 Hertz, a musical C. That is universal. That also happens to be in the alpha brain frequency range experienced during meditation. From that, the Daoists and Yogis have mapped frequencies of color, sound, and myriad other properties onto the five elements and the meridians, as well as to the chakra system. For example: The root chakra in yoga, located at the perineum, is associated with fire, physical needs, the tone C, and the color red. In acupuncture and five element theory, it is also an end point on the conception vessel—which runs up the front of the body through all the chakras—and is a reservoir for the yin meridians. The color red in five element theory is also associated with the fire element and the small intestine (yang organ) and heart (yin organ) (Kaptchuk, 1983, p. 53). Each one of the yin and yang meridians that are connected through the conception and governing vessels is mapped to its own color associations, sounds, emotions, and much more.

Modern medicine also analyzes frequency of different aspects of the body's flesh and bones through technologies such as CAT, MRI, and PET scans which measure spectral energy (Lipton, 2005, pp. 114–15). On the molecular and atomic levels, new mass spectromic scanners are now on the market that can identify the molecular components in both organic or nonorganic samples, from blood samples to astroturf. Even DNA are capable of sending out a range of frequencies and are an essential source of light and biophoton emissions (McTaggart, 2008, p. 48).

Colors, as seen in auras, also correlate to frequency ranges. For example, blue is 250–275 Hz, green 250–475 Hz, yellow 500–700 Hz, orange 950–1050 Hz, red 1000–1200 Hz, violet 1000–2000 Hz, white 1100–2000 Hz (Brennan, 1987, p. 33). Each color is associated with personality traits and health status.

Frequencies of emotions and levels of consciousness are also measurable. David Hawkins, using a kinesthesiologic muscle testing technique, established his own scale from 200 to 1,000 to define states of consciousness. On the low end of the scale are shame (20), guilt (30), and apathy (50). The scale then moves up through grief (75), fear (100), desire (125), anger (150), and pride (175). Things shift around 200 to more positive qualities such as courage, neutrality (250), willingness (310), acceptance (350), and reason (400). On the upper end of the scale one finds love (500), joy (540), peace (600) and enlightenment (700–1000) (Hawkins, 2002, p. 75). These higher level emotions correspond to LeShan's description of nonquantitative and continuous consciousness—or "attaining the Dao" (Kohn, 2010, p. 60).

When Daoist texts refer to the golden elixir they are referring to a state of constancy and immutability at the upper levels of this scale. This higher state of consciousness "manifests in the golden hue the adept's body emits after he or she fully completes the practice" (Ho, 2018). Cross culturally, this is also depicted by the golden haloes around saintly figures such as Mary and Jesus in Christian art.

The Wen-Tzu commentary on Laozi from circa 100 BCE also evokes the five elements and delineates levels of personal development.

> In ancient times the Master of the Center said that the sky has five directions, the earth has five elements, music has five notes, things have five flavors, matter has five primary colors, people have five positions. Thus there are twenty-five kinds of people between sky and earth.

The highest are the spiritual people, real people, people of the Way, perfected people, and sages.

Next are people with virtue, wise people, knowing people, good people, and discerning people.

In the middle are fair people, faithful people, trustworthy people, just people, and courteous people.

Next are scholars, craftspeople, foresters, farmers, and merchants.

Lowest are people without individuality, servile people, stupid people, people who are like lumps of meat, and petty people.

The difference between the highest five and the lowest five types is like the difference between humans and oxen or horses (Cleary, 1991, p. 90).

Taken altogether, there is a frequency aspect to everything within our sensory experience and beyond. Taiji practice entails refining one's qi and returning to one's highest essence (*jing*) through forms and meditation practices to attain pure mind/spirit (*shen*). Thus, the ability to see light via auras and perceive high pitched sound or emotions in another person suggest heightened inner stillness and alignment to Dao. Opening to qi allows one's life force frequency to interact with the body container of the bones, emotions, body fluids, tissue, and the spaces that bind it all together. Slowly the vibration of these parts can synergistically align to the fundamental overtone of the earth[7]. This attunement to the natural world is fundamental to Daoist internal mastery (Liping, 2019, p. 35).

In small groups, like a chamber music ensemble, we vibrate in relation not only to the earth but to each other. Individuals share that root frequency but have different sets of overtones. When people

---

[7] Should you favor a more universal perspective, Kepler's 1619 Harmonices Mundi uses elliptical orbits of the planets and their velocities to define the harmony of planetary motion. A sound realization of these equations was recorded by Yale professors, John Rogers and Willie Ruff. It was included by Carl Sagan on the Golden Record for the Voyager Mission (Rodgers and Ruff).

are compatible, they blend and grow stronger together, like a well-tuned string quartet. When two sources, such as lovers or soulmates, vibrate at the same level or complementary levels in consonance, their combined overtone series yields a shimmery vibrancy and larger sound. A psychic once described that phenomenon to me as the "tuning fork effect" (a tuning fork vibrates silently until it contacts a resonator which amplifies and, therefore, audibly releases its song). Lipton describes the phenomenon as "constructive interferences or good vibes," (Lipton, 2005, pp. 120–1). Likewise, two people who dislike each other, or are in conflict, do not merge into consonance but remain out of tune or in well-tuned dissonance. Maybe they just do not do much for each other, such as a tuba and violin attempting to form a duet. Or maybe they clash outright as their upper overtones interact in a dissonant way.

With awareness, you may become more tolerant as you open to all and more easily find entrainment with people, but you are not going to find that luscious tuning fork effect with everyone you meet. Consonance will be common. Dissonance, too, will be common, making pure consonance a delightful blessing. Acceptance of both the consonant and dissonant as well as learning appropriate responses is part of the taiji path as it maneuvers us out of the realm of the mind and into the interplay of energies. This is particularly apparent in push hands practice that emphasizes listening and neutralizing. Classmates, like meditators in a retreat, who give up a bit of their individual selves in doing the form in order to stay with the group, may find a powerful qi that is impossible to replicate the rest of the week on one's own.

The metaphor of resonance with Dao is not just a western imposition. The second-century-BCE text, *Huainanzi*, presents the same analogy.

> When the lute tuner strikes the kung note [on one instrument], the kung note [on the other instrument] responds: when he plucks the chiao note [on one instrument], the chiao note [on the other instrument] vibrates. This results from having corresponding musical notes in mutual harmony.

Now, [let us assume that] someone changes the tuning of one string in such a way that it does not match any of the five notes, and by striking it sets all twenty-five strings resonating. In this case there has as yet been no differentiation as regards sound; it just happens that that [sound] which governs all musical notes has been evoked.

Thus, he who is merged with Supreme Harmony is beclouded as if dead-drunk, and drifts about in its midst in sweet contentment, unaware how he came there; engulfed in pure delight as he sinks to the depths; benumbed as he reaches the end, he is as if he had not yet begun to emerge from his origin. This is called the Great Merging (Le Blanc, 1985).

However valuable sensitivity to supersensory phenomena are to the taiji player as a learning tool, the classics repeatedly forewarn us not to be waylaid by mystical ephemera in pursuit of this "Great Merging."

The old man [Lao Tzu] said, "When the spirit is projected too soon, before it is purged of mundane shadows, it is called the dark spirit. When it emerges, one may see white light in some form, in which case the spirit is emerging from the eyes; or one may hear the sound of bells, cymbals, and pipes, in which case the spirit is emerging from the ears. Because the light energy is not strong enough, it cannot break through the Celestial Pass, and therefore goes off on side roads, whichever is easiest. After emerging, it also roams around blissfully, through the streets and alleys, to the rivers and up the mountains. It can only take form, it cannot multiply form, it can only travel in the human realm, it cannot fly and transmute. On a sunny midsummer day, the dark spirit will fear and flee the sun; so even though it has something of the air of immortals about it, still it is not beyond the realm of ghosts. —Commentary on Sun Bu-er by Chen Yingning (Cleary, 2000, pp. 430–1).

Mind and the Etheric Body

Liu [Cao] writes: "if the basic energy is not stabilized, the spirit is insecure. Let insects eat away the roots of a tree, and the leaves dry up. Stop talking about mucus, saliva, semen, and blood—when you get to the basis and find out the original source, they are all the same. When has this thing ever had a fixed location? It changes according to the time, according to mind and ideas. In the body it becomes perspiration when feeling heat, in the eyes it becomes tears when feeling sadness, in the genitals it becomes semen when feeling attention, in the nose it becomes mucus when feeling cold. It flows all over, moistening the whole body; ultimately it is nothing more than the spiritual water.

—(Cleary, 1999, p. 346)

In taiji, our practice focuses first on the body, strengthening the organs, calming the nervous system, and striving for our physical alignment between heaven and earth. When our skeletons do fall into alignment, the electrophysiological connections and nervous system face less resistance and greater flow. People often first discover qi in their physical bodies through feelings of buzzing or fullness. In the mind, meanwhile, they often begin to experience clarity, calmness, and easing of emotions.

Emotions are also manifestations of energy, and the mentally healthier the person, the more serene they are likely to be. Regardless, people describe releases of emotion, sometimes through tears or laughter. Such startling changes in demeanor, mood, and personality are a wakeup call to many that this practice is something to pay attention to as emotions are key touchpoints of the egoic mind and a manifestation of our sense of self.

Mind, paradoxically, may be the hardest part of the body, mind, spirit trilogy to get our heads around, because we really don't know what mind is. That said, the evidence of what it is not, is mounting. It is not the brain. It is not the creator of thought. In fact, guidance from accounts of near death experiences suggests its residence is not restricted to the brain. And yet in this postliterate information age, it is where most of what we believe to be "us" resides.

Functionally, mind can be seen as the bridge between body and spirit, the connective tissue between the slower matter of our physical bodies and the light of our spiritual bodies. It is also a garbage dump where emotion, thoughts, reactions, desires, fears, joy, anticipation, and expectation lurk. It is the general-in-command that allows us to function and survive on this earth—directing us to eat and care for our bodies, to work to earn the resources to have something to eat, and to teach our progeny as we have been taught.

It is that general, sometimes emerging as ego, that can tip things out of balance with its self-importance. All nondual spiritual traditions work to quiet the mind, allowing balance to pervade. In balance, our bodies are healthy, our minds are calm, and our spirits are strong. In taiji practice, the manifestations of qi that people experience in this realm often lay the foundation for spiritual and mystical growth.

Chris' statement, "I feel happy when I do the form," is really quite a profound discovery as it reflects a change in consciousness and emotional vibration. If all that we know or experience boils down to energy, then it makes sense that through practice our discernment should become subtler. In the physical body, which we know to be comprised of atoms and molecules, it is possible to more than imagine infinitely small parts in constant motion. As relaxation takes hold, and systems in the body and mind start settling down, a calmer awareness comes into play as the physical body and mind let go of tension and anxiety.

Moving past the body and mind into the auric layers, things are every bit as dynamic, and the emanating energy is palpable to many senses. Aura frequency is revealed to sight through color or the perception of shimmering waves, brightness on a hot summer's day, or even a mirage. To the ears, frequency is revealed through overtones and timbre. Expanded perception may include not only high and low tones but clairaudient voices. In touch, frequency is revealed as the sense of tingling, static, gooiness, vibrancy, or radiancy moving through one's hands or body.

It is in the aura where many energetic healers and psychics work, using their sense of touch, intuition, or sight. It is the information highway of our essence, reflecting and revealing truths that we may not outwardly acknowledge. The aura's kaleidoscopic array of color reveals our overall state of being, illness, and changes in mood or thought. It is a level where you cannot mask your true emotions, hide behind armoring behaviors, or pretend to have control.

People experience auras in many ways, but for now, it is illustrative to talk about them in terms of color. Those who see colors, or who have had a Kirlian photograph taken, see varying hues and intensity. Barbara Brennan cites studies mapping out the frequency of the colors in *Hands of Light*. Black and brown vibrate at the low end of the spectrum, and, moving through the rainbow, the frequency rises until reaching white, vibrating at over 1100 Hz (Brennan, 1987). That same energy, to the psychic, reveals a panorama of past life and subconscious information, including passions, fears, personality traits, and states of being. To a healer, the aura may reveal all of that or simply an area of pain.

It was through push hands that I first consciously experienced energy on this level. When the barriers broke down, I could feel the intent of a push before it was triggered and the path of energy moving through my body. This sensitivity quickly developed to the point that I felt as if I knew the essence of a person beyond words within minutes with more truth than I could have after years of acquaintance or intimacy. That we can sense fear, pain, joy, or peace through the hypersenses, or the paranormal, was revelatory.

Aura readers, like astrologists, have mapped out personality traits and correlations with the rainbow. Green is the color of healers; blue is the color of nurturers; tan is the province of engineers and analytic thinkers; purple is a mark of spirituality and creativity, and yellow is indicative of joy and nonattachment. Intensity and shade vary from person to person, day-to-day, and minute to minute as inner processes change. People often display a combination of colors.

For example, my usual aura has elements of violet, blue, and green. Sitting in a post migraine stupor one afternoon, my son walked down the stairs and shuddered, "I hate it when Mom's aura is brown."

Another day he informed me that I turned brown when I was angry (an adept diversion from the teen conflict triggering that anger). Lynn recalls not recognizing an acquaintance at a party when her aura was altered in color and shape by cancer.

In the Daoist tradition, immortality is understood as higher level consciousness. Mental ease and longer life are byproducts of the practices as the individual frees himself from stress and tension (Cleary, 2000, p. 307). By transforming and refining one's qi, through meditation and trance training, healing exercises, and diet, one overcomes the pull of the mind and flows with nature, in mystical rapture with the Dao.

> While the ultimate goal of Daoist practice is this transformation to transcendence or immortality, practitioners have always embraced all the different levels and increased their mental acuity and spiritual subtlety to find a closer connection to Dao and enhance quality of life. Mental health relevant to living in the world appears dominantly on the middle level, where the individual is still fully part of the world but his or her toxic emotions are transformed into virtues and self and mind are lessened to again let body-form and spirit shine forth in their original purity. (Kohn, 2011, p. 19)

Let us return to this middle level.

Leyla recalls that she used to get very depressed and have low energy levels. Taiji and qigong have given her tools to come back out of that state.

> The more I let go of constriction and control, and the more the energy flows through my body, the more there's some kind of impersonal energy. I'm really recognizing the difference between ego and how rigid that is, versus this flowing kind of connection between the qi in the body and the mind—like personal spirit. There's a connection there. And I'm just beginning to discover that relationship. The more I let go, the more something else takes over and to be able to leave me this body and doing things in a way that's in alignment and harmony with this life.

In fact, changes in mind are a critical part of the martial arts training. Roosevelt Gainey found that it took him about six years to switch from relying on muscular strength to using internal strength. "Internal martial arts *is* the mind, not the body. Internal martial arts *is* training the mind, not training the body. [You] use the body to free the mind. But once your mind is free you have complete movement."

Discussing the stages of qi discovery, after the usual tingling in the fingers, Grandmaster William Chen explains that the next stage is a whole body connection to the energy, emanating from the ground and moving through the foot and up through the body. "It took me about 45 years. I finally found Three Nails, connecting the foot to the ground. The toes also function as a brain, as does the thumb. I consider [it] like three brains. If you have headaches, you don't massage your head. You massage your toe or thumb." The naturalness of this is such that in its simplicity, people miss it, says Chen. Yet if you use kinesthetic muscle testing to objectively evaluate Chen's technique, you will find a gentle press of the big toe creates very strong tensegrity in the body.

The next stage, says Chen, is to develop a whole body connection to the energy through practice of the form. Using the taiji form as a meditation, concentrating exclusively on his movement, he centers himself while shutting down mind chatter.

> Exhaling will help clear your mind. Once the exhale clears up your mind, then you start to inhale. Inhaling, your mind starts waking up. And when your mind wakes up you tell your mind, or tell your body, what you want to do. So when you're shaping the posture in that minute, you're waking up. The energy automatically flows wherever you want it flow.
>
> … When you relax, your mind changes. … When mind decreases [qi goes] all the way down to the base. Exhaling helps two things. One, is clear up your mind. Two, is go with gravity so everything goes down. When your mind wakes up, that's the compression of the energies starting to come up.

Such rising and falling energies of mind can set the stage for significant personal growth. Don Miller reflects:

> This is something that didn't happen immediately, but over thirty years and is still continuing, but it took the edge off what otherwise had been an excessively yang personality and body type. I think the direction I was going was more reactive, more angry, more unyielding than was probably optimal for me in the life that I've chosen to live. So I often say the taiji has kept me out of jail and/or kept me from killing someone or getting killed. And I think that's true because ... the philosophical idea in Daoism that when yin or yang reaches its limit—when anything reaches its limit—first of all it's bad, and it starts to turn into its opposite, or it starts to fall apart. Taiji enables you to round the curve or turn back the other way before you drive over the edge of the cliff. And it has served that purpose for me thousands of times.

Roosevelt Gainey witnessed patterns of profound changes in countless students with different personalities, different religions, and different taiji styles. Among them all, he begins to notice more self-awareness and self-confidence.

> I tell people you have to get your family to do this with you. Or in eight months, they're not going to know you. *Because you evolve.*
>
> Stuck is one of the causes of major sickness. You can trace almost every sickness back to emotional imbalance. Not just imbalance, but ... If you're angry too much you cause a lot of different things. If you're angry or depressed, certain illnesses will be forthcoming from your standing in that state of mind [and] energy disruption that keeps going through your system.

One student of Rosie's was a particular standout. A developmentally challenged boy with the cognitive capacity of a five-year-old, arrived at Rosie's school at age fourteen wanting to learn martial arts.

> He couldn't see from here to that wall. He was almost blind. I made him start standing. And he would ask me, "Teach, how long I been standing?" I said, "Five minutes." An hour [had] passed. He had no sense of time. He had no short-term memory; hardly any long-term memory. After two years, I took him over to the Circle of Masters in Jersey and he defeated the top, top fighter of the east coast—beat him like he was a baby. Then I got him *Hooked on Phonics*—had him teach himself to read. He got his high school diploma.

At age thirty-nine, says Rosie, he tested normally on I.Q. tests, was working, and had two beautiful normal little girls.

Changes in levels of consciousness and brain states are not usually so dramatic, but they are not uncommon among people who practice neigong, qigong, and various meditation postures. Taken to an extreme, however, unguided practice can result in the kind of kundalini psychosis described earlier. But openness to higher energies also leads people to big breakthroughs, and longtime practitioners mostly learn to integrate that energy and operate from a higher level of consciousness.

Micaela, a college sophomore, describes the transitional state so many go through before integrating the energy:

> It's like taking lots and lots of drugs and not being able to control it. I go really, really deep. One time, I actually was moved by another force. That was kind of trippy. When I do the form on a daily basis, I feel like I'm walking taller and that the world is brighter and not as condensed. It gives me the feeling of expanse.

Carolyn recalls her first awareness of qi as a "floaty, bubbly, gooey, gummy feeling." She also found herself wanting to shake her head slowly and wave her hands, Miss America style. She was immediately taken in by the meditative relaxation, her feeling of being cleansed, and the brighter feeling the practice brought to her day and, in time, her heightened sensitivity.

Deena, a relative beginner in her middle years recognizes that "I'm more aligned. I'm calmer. I'm not so quick to react, although I still react quickly. I don't get tensed up. But I have a little bit more of a gentle quality about me now. I go slower when situations are arising."

Diana, a long time student reflects,

> I feel that I have more confidence in myself. I dance better. I'm less inhibited in my own body when I dance so therefore it's much more enjoyable. I'm lighter and happier when I'm in what I would call a taiji state or attitude—I'm much more alive, but calm. It's a calm alertness, a calm aliveness, but it's very definitely more alive. And I'm more fun to be around.

Eleanor, the taiji star of a nearby senior center, did not start classes until she was in her sixties. A Polish immigrant, through the nine years of her study she recognizes many changes in herself.

> I open up to people. I'm more outgoing. If somebody said to me nine years ago, "Do taiji here," I would head out the door. So I'm much more open and thank God for that. I don't know if I could handle my husband with his seizures if I hadn't been in taiji. And this is my therapy.

Chenoa acknowledges lack of boundaries between people and greater awareness of others' emotional states in addition to increased focus and calm. "I'm really aware of other people's energy. I can feel other people's emotions, and I think this used to happen to me before but I wouldn't know it was coming from someone else."

Learning to receive qi has been a challenge for Chenoa. It is hard to just let it be without reacting to others people's problems and, so, she sometimes just retreats. One day, at a workshop she felt the disparity between a man's polite, outward demeanor yet sexually threatening energy. "I felt really sick and disgusted afterwards like as if he had raped me or something." Like many women who listen to their sixth sense, Chenoa did not stick around to explore this man's intentions.

Maggie Newman has had similar experiences with people whose energy is so aggressive that she felt the urge to disconnect from it.

> Sometimes I think one needs a shield to keep negative energy, or aggressive energy from coming in. But that's because I'm not enlightened in that area. If I were, then that energy could just go through me, and it wouldn't exhaust me. When you're around that, it's very hard not to react back. So you have the principles of taiji there. Taiji is a great tool.

On the flip side, being in the presence of others can also be inspiring. Jonathan Shear relates many experiences of entering a state of transcendence merely by being in the presence of others in that realm of consciousness.

One time at Berkeley, a Zen master was walking by while Shear was having a conversation. When the master walked within about fifty feet, Shear felt himself shift.

> I was new to that stuff. I'd go through the motions of continuing my conversation. He'd walk right by, and I'd turn and I'd say, "Hello, Mori." Or he'd say, "Hello, Jonathan." I'd go through the motions of that. When he'd pass it would be on the same distance on the other side, and I'd be back in a normal consciousness.

Shear also describes being around Maharishi in the 1960s and when coming within thirty or forty feet from him, feeling like being on a psychedelic. One time, he sat in a lecture hall with about a thousand other people, well back in the hall. Maharishi was discussing consciousness as a cyclic wave. A wave, explains Shear, has a base, and crests and falls over. But as the wave expands its base, it takes on the power of the whole motion. Having a degree in pure math and some background in physics, he was trying to puzzle that out—what it really means for a wave to take on the power of the ocean—meanwhile the lecture continued. "There I was, maybe five hundred people back. And there he is looking right in my eyes, right in the middle of giving his lecture, and saying "It's *just* an analogy.""

Shear conferred with many people who had been around Maharishi for some length of time, and learned that this often happened. Maharishi's lectures were woven together by his responding to thoughts that people in the audience were hung up on. "He looks right in your eyes, and he's [answering] your question." David Hawkins claims that such entrainment is a common experience for devotees in the presence of teachers whose energy fields calibrate at 550 [love] and over (Hawkins, 2002, p. 262).

In martial arts settings, Shear describes several instances of transcendence. In the push hands experience, he says, one is usually focused on catching somebody, or being caught. However, when one lets go and gets into the flow, it is possible to preserve the feel of the flow in the midst of the match [*wu wei*]. As a result, one inevitably plays better.

Likewise, a taiji teacher's hand guiding a correction in one's back or hips, can be more effective than any verbal instruction as the correction comes with embodied energy. Sometimes described as "transmission by touch," these lessons reinforce the value of live interaction as a teaching tool as some lessons one just can't get through a book or video.

Recalling an encounter during his student days, Shear describes feeling space.

> [Y]ou could feel and see it, and it was alive and all the objects, the people in it, were just sort of floating like these big rocks. The Master's teacher came to the U.S. to do some advanced stuff... He was a seventh degree in Judo, which is inordinately high, and he was the Japanese Minister of Education. I was racked up with injuries at the time. And I'm standing there just watching and [the Master] didn't speak any English at all, and he starts coming up to me ... and all of a sudden, boom, I'm in this altered state. Everything is glowing, and his face becomes smooth—filling maybe, 70 or 80 percent of my visual field.

... That next day, I'm talking to my teacher, and he comes up and says "Oh, Shimizo. You're a good researcher." That stunned me. How could this guy know that? Up until then my whole background—I grew up on—my father was the guy who started chemotherapy for cancer ... I grew up being trained as a researcher.

Effects on one's consciousness, however, are not always so dramatic. Ken Van Sickle:

Someone once asked Cheng Man Ching, does taiji change your character? He said, "probably not, that's very, very difficult." I was surprised by that because I had already noticed change in some peoples' character and since then have seen drastic change in peoples' character. I think it was sort of like covering his ass, like "don't expect your character to change."

The first thing I see in people is their balance gets better. Their leg strength gets better, and these are all physical things. Great, your balance and your leg strength get better; you know your heart is in better shape right away.

Then I see their manner softening along with that. Then when people get further into it, and especially the push hands, I see their manner changing in their relationships a little bit—with some people more than others. The hardest problems are the men—strong men. Young, strong men. They have a hard time not getting into the combat of it and wanting to be the one to win. That really stops them. The women's problem is that they don't want to use any kind of strength, even the correct kind. So they both have their problems. But the men's problem is usually bigger because many of them, in fact like 60 percent never really end up being able to do taiji while they're doing push hands. They always resort to struggling.

... Taiji people always seem a lot younger, all other things being equal, than other people of the same age.

How is it that a physical practice such as taiji can create a sense of wellbeing, balance, and serenity? Don Miller:

> Where it leads is where taiji wants you to go, which is that you can relax more physically, mentally, and emotionally. That you feel connected to the earth, sometimes in a shamanic way. You feel grounded. And the upper body, or I would say the rest of the body, including the legs, if you get that far, the body is willing to let go of a lot of its residual tension, and soften and to move in all kinds of ways that otherwise it wouldn't want to move in. It makes all the stuff that they talk about in taiji in terms of the body softening and being flexible and being, well supple ...

> Supple, and all of which I view as getting fear out of your body, out of your tissues, out of your cells. There's residual fear, and then there's the fear that occurs in response to some perceived threat. And both of those are reduced by having root. Root is kind of the antidote to fear. If you really have a lot of root, you cannot have a fear reaction. You cannot have the fight or flight reaction. Root is really an energetic phenomenon. It's not a physical phenomenon of people with strong legs. It has nothing to do with strong legs, although it's often associated with a lot of legwork, or stance work, but ultimately it really is an energetic phenomenon where, your energy body shifts downward or it grows downward.

> Fear and excessive reactivity to anything we refer to as the qi coming up. But if your root is really deep, your qi can't come up. Not to the degree that will imbalance you, that will make your top heave, energetically, or excessively reactive or prone to anger, fear, and other destabilizing emotions. I don't include grief or sadness in those because they're not in the fear camp.

Just as the world's great religions will never settle who has seen the Truth, so goes the taiji experience. However, many a taiji satori has been triggered by changes in consciousness through this practice. Some reflect gradual shifts in perception while others can be described as mystical or spiritual. All are valid signs of incremental alignment with Dao.

111

The Mystical Realm of Greater Sensual Perception

The old man [Lao Tzu] said, "When the spirit is projected too soon, before it is purged of mundane shadows, it is called the dark spirit. When it emerges, one may see white light in some form, in which case the spirit is emerging from the eyes; or one may hear the sound of bells, cymbals, and pipes, in which case the spirit is emerging from the ears. Because the light energy is not strong enough, it cannot break through the Celestial Pass, and therefore goes off on side roads, whichever is easiest. After emerging, it also roams around blissfully, through the streets and alleys, to the rivers and up the mountains. It can only take form, it cannot multiply form, it can only travel in the human realm, it cannot fly and transmute. On a sunny midsummer day, the dark spirit will fear and flee the sun; so even though it has something of the air of immortals about it, still it is not beyond the realm of ghosts."

—Commentary on Sun Bu-er by Chen Yingning
(Cleary, 2000, pp. 434–5)

Mystical insights at the root of Daoist tradition—as expressed through Laozi, Zhuangzi, Ancestor Lü Yan, Sun Bu-er, and others—include, presumably, the roots of five element theory. Tsou Yen first described both yin yang and five phases in the second century BCE (Roth, 1999, pp. 21–2). Cycles of generation and destruction through the fire, water, wood, metal, and earth elements are used to explain our natural surroundings as well as health. Each element is associated with organs of the body, emotions, colors, smells, sounds, animals, personality type, etc… Michael Stanley-Baker writes about the medieval Upper Clarity school's purposeful integration of visualization into both massage and daoyin (precursor to qigong) to move beyond merely curing disease and improving general health and toward mystical states of consciousness (Stanley-Baker, 2012).

The qualities mapped out in the five element cycle are not the work of linear minds. Rather it is knowledge acquired by acute observation, intuition, higher vision, and supersensory perception of the mystic. Tapping into this paradigm, cultivation of qi through taiji, qigong, and alchemic practices are means for the individual to bring these elements into balance on one's own.

Like the Buddhists, ancient Daoists recognized that mystical insights are a byproduct of higher levels of consciousness. While the Buddhists keep things in perspective by dismissing illusory phenomenon, the Daoists caution against doggedly pursuing extrasensory practices. Ancestor Lü labeled these sometimes rather enjoyable, and sometimes rather dangerous, byproducts of primordial energy "deviant practices," (Cleary, 2000, p. 93).

> The Great Way is like a level road. If you do not proceed to traverse the level road by way of true consciousness, you fall into sidetracks. When people get mixed up in any of the countless cults, even if they are admonished they can rarely wake up, and even if there is true guidance they do not follow it. Even if causeless consciousness, consciousness of the future, consciousness of sound and form, and consciousness of the past are all forgotten, still if the consciousness of personal knowledge is kept you will be lost after all— Ancestor Lü (Cleary, 2000).

It is not uncommon for taiji players to develop supersensory capabilities, and, indeed, such attunement to subtler energies can also be viewed as the dissolving of barriers between subject and object. Sensing an object's energy field, either visually or through feeling, as it moves from lower to higher frequencies, or perhaps solid to vaporous matter, one is less and less able to differentiate where an object's edges are. In that diffuse space, the energy of two objects is apt to mingle and exchange information. In addition to feeling as if one is being caressed by grace, people also describe how difficult it is to learn to operate in this world with so much frequency flowing through the body.

For those finding themselves in mystical states seeing auras, hearing extreme high or low frequencies, feeling energies, or developing psychic capabilities, such "deviant" or tangential practices, can be useful stepping stones.

It is worth bearing in mind that auras are not just a figment of the mystic mind. Yale neuroanatomist Harold Burr (1889–1973) "discovered electrical fields around all sorts of organisms from molds, to salamanders and frogs, to humans. Changes in the electrical charges appeared to correlate with growth, sleep, regeneration, light, water, storms, the development of cancer—even the waxing and waning of the moon. For instance, in his experiments with plant seedlings, he discovered electrical fields which resembled the eventual adult plant" (McTaggart, 2008, p. 48). The groundbreaking neuro researcher, Karl Pribram, found evidence that discernment of smell, taste, and hearing, in fact, operate by analyzing frequencies (McTaggart, 2008, p. 87), and, today, one can have a Kirlian photo taken of one's aura at any psychic fair.

My own exposure to higher frequency information through auras and touch has greatly shaped and reframed my view of reality to embrace the porousness of our world. As the concrete solidity of subjects and objects viewed from the vessel of my own form started to disintegrate, I could extend beyond my body to connect with another across hundreds of miles in a remote healing session. In meditation, the venerable maple tree and I were really not distinct, but fuzzy concentrations of coagulated energy. So are individuals. Psychics transcend the space between people, spirits, and past lives, connecting across the common sphere of unlimited consciousness, and they are able to interpret paranormal information through their senses.

Bruce Lipton points out that alpha wave activity is equated with calm consciousness. "While most of our senses, such as eyes, ears, and nose, observe the outer world, consciousness resembles a sense organ that behaves like a mirror reflecting back the inner workings of the body's own cellular community; it is an awareness of self." That sense of self, however, is signaled by perception of stimuli or frequency through the cell membranes (Lipton, 2005, p. 190).

The variety of ways people receive and interpret mystical information is informed by the size, shape, personality, and subconscious of the receiver. Interpretation of energy through paranormal sensation is also where many enter the land of faith. The feeling of truth that may accompany any incident reinforces conviction in that experience as a window to higher consciousness. The forms in which psychic information are received are custom fit to our strengths and weaknesses and shaped by our cultural mythologies just as our dreams are. In his extensive analysis of shamanic visioning, Holger Kalweit explains,

> There is no objectivity in psychic space, just as there is none in the material realm. In Einstein's universe, space and time are functions dependent on the observer. Similarly, a culturally-conditioned psyche will interpret both the outer and inner world subjectively and in accordance with its own frame of reference points. Nevertheless, behind these culturally diversified interpretations of reality a number of common features are beginning to emerge (Kalweit, 1988, p. 124).

For David Chandler, all five senses are portals to higher frequencies, but touch was the vehicle for his first taiji inspired satori:

> When I was finished with class, I walked outside and walked down the stairs. I grabbed the banister, and I felt the banister like I'd never felt anything before in my life. The sense of touch was so incredibly enhanced at this point. I felt power going through my body in such a way that I could take that banister and go grrpppppp, rip it off the wall and poke it through the ceiling and walls. And I went, "but don't do that."
> ... It was this incredible awakening of the senses that manifested first in the sense of touch. The tactile awareness was extraordinarily enhanced. ...I was already feeling relaxed. I was feeling buzzy, I was buzzing in my fingers and hands. This was the sense of power that I didn't want to test fully, but certainly wanted to play with. It was like suddenly going from bicycle to combustion machine in the body.

Shortly thereafter, I had a similar experience. I rode my bike home and was hungry. I was going to make a sandwich, grabbed a bottle of milk, put it on the table, and put some other stuff on the table. Then later I turned and reached for the bottle of milk, and I just touched it. I reached; I touched it; it went Boom! And it went right against this wall and went spssh... the whole wall was covered with milk! And I just went, "I want to know how to do that again." Because all I did was touch it and it flew. And I went, "I'm getting it." This is qi. I just released jing from my body." I didn't have the terminology, but I had the experience.

David is somewhat unusual in that all of his senses were enhanced through his opening to qi and that he developed synesthesia as well.

Oftentimes today, we'll be out someplace, and I'll go "phone is ringing" and people will go, I don't hear anything. "Run, the phone is ringing." And, they'll get to the door and go "Ohhhh" because they can hardly believe it. Sense of hearing becomes very acute, I find.

Sense of sight, seeing beyond seeing, is, I think, one of the keys to what happens when you play taiji. I think for some people it functions as auras, I see that. That's not where I go all the time. I'll look at someone and go "Oooh, a golden light around them." But what happens is, if I look to the side and spend a moment then that kind of thing occurs. It becomes seeing that becomes much more visceral. You feel the seeing. So it all goes back to the sense of touch. You see it; you feel it. You smell it; you feel it.

My sense of smell tends to be pretty heightened as well.

When I first started to experience qi, it immediately became something for me that I knew was on a spiritual path as well as practicing something that was physical—had physical demeanor to it. The physical demeanor was one thing, but the internal awakening that was happening was outstripping everything.

116

In addition to cultural conditioning, multiple intelligences or aptitudes also play into how people gain insight to higher energies (Gardner, 2008, pp. 8–21).

David's synesthesia makes sense in that he was trained as an actor. In order to portray a character, an actor embraces all the characteristics of that personality shedding his sense of self in the process. To become another, he has to listen to the quality of voice, accent, and linguistic mannerisms, and he feels the emotions and thoughts of that identity to make the lines convincing. It makes sense that in his taiji awakening, he became more open to all the senses, and they become indistinct.

An illustrator, Lynn, sees vividly colored auras. Trained as a musician, I am most sensitive to sound and the feel of sound. And like most people who start to experience frequencies through one sense, others start opening as well, although maybe not to the extent of our trained sense.

Micaela's supersensory hearing ability has been difficult to synthesize. Not only can she hear her own body's bones creaking and muscles stretching, but she is hyperaware of others. "That's actually the hardest part of my life because it's not in a good way. I think it started when I was nine. Stuff like chewing gum and chewy crunchy things bother me. Someone chewing gum during a test will drive into me like nails."

In my everyday life, the incoherent noise of a crowd or electrical amplification are quick paths to a headache, and a barking dog feels like the stab of a knife. However, on a silent retreat when I was physically and emotionally wide open, sneezes and coughs in the meditation hall could be felt approaching from fifty feet away, passing through my body, and exiting through the other side. Dissipating into the distance, the experience took on mystical qualities. On that same retreat, from the sound of the gong at the end of a sitting I could hear overtones two octaves beyond what I normally distinguish and a rather angelic tinnitus was a steady companion to sitting with the breath. Needless to say, my reacclimation, or retraction, into a populated electronic world was slow.

Maggie Newman experiences sound on the low end of the spectrum in connection to taiji practice.

> It's not a sound of a muscle or anything. It wasn't high pitched. It was deeper. It was sort of like hearing chanting of some kind, but it's not a chant. It's just a sound. I think it's just a physiological thing—almost like an instrument is finely tuned or something in nature that make sounds because of the wind.

As Jonathan Shear pointed out, any nondual meditation or taiji practice can refine one's ability to receive subtle information. That can be transcendent, either in one's consciousness or perception. Years ago Shear spent nearly a year at a meditation retreat in Switzerland. One day he walked outside and heard incredibly beautiful music. He thought somebody was walking outside with a boom box. Imagine his surprise in discovering that he was listening to the groaning squeak of a rusty door hinge.

Don Miller's experiences reflect the shamanic immersion that for him is integral to taiji. (More on shamanist shadings to come.) Opening the senses for him opens a conduit for communication from the spirit world. One time, he was taking a martial arts knife fighting seminar with a friend. Returning from the lunch break, listening to the radio while driving, Don pulled into the left-hand turn lane.

> Just as I shifted into the turn lane the guy on the radio said, "Don, always remember to use your turn signal indicator when changing lanes. And then he went right back to the news, or the weather or whatever it was. But he interrupted what he was saying at that moment when I was turning, without using my turn signal indicator, by the way, and it went back to the news.

> Now, the first thing I did, because I know that people hear things, is without prejudicing him, I just asked Matthew, "Tell me exactly what you just heard." And he said, "I heard the guy on the radio say, "Don, always remember to use your turn signal indicator when changing lanes." I said, "That's what I heard."

We were both pretty stunned by this. And I thought about it a lot and am absolutely convinced that this came on my radio; it was on my radio. I don't believe it was anyone else's radio. I don't believe that the actual guy doing that show at that moment gave that message out to everyone in LA who was listening to that station, but that somehow, I can't even hazard the details of this, but somehow I was being given a message from some other entity, dimension, guardian angel—I have no idea what exactly—through the radio. But for some reason the message was also audible to my friend, which puts it in a different category than just hearing a voice in your head…

In addition to practicing taiji, Tom M. also works within the shamanic tradition of visualization and is open to receiving information through unusual pathways.

It's not a clear picture but it's almost like something being projected inside. When I do hear things it is more just knowing I heard it. One time, a little over a year ago, I did hear a voice. I had been reading a book on channeling and I was sitting on a subway platform on a bench and I was almost totally alone. I heard this voice say, "What now, Tom?" I turned around both ways and nobody was around.

Like David, Sarah experiences energy through all her senses and has an unusual sense of hearing, especially in the high frequency range. She is sensitive to the energy of crystals and other people, and she can see energy in different ways. Psychic, even as a child, she says, "I always thought it was just part of being a hypersensitive. All my senses are off a little bit." When she was young, she played with seeing the colors of auras but now does not normally see color. "I see variations of light frequency. I see zigzag lines; I see different textures. It's like seeing music."

Aura watching can be remarkably moving and even entertaining, like watching live art in motion. Sarah loves go to the taiji school and just watch.

The best class to see energy is the taiji conditioning class. It's fun because everybody's juiced, but they're all concentrating on the same thing. And you see the same patterns between people. I might see shapes sometimes, like I might see an hourglass kind of figure of energy going up somebody's back. You might see that same thing on each person. It might be a little heavier on the bottom on one, or a little more diffused on the top of another. Or it might not be there for somebody else who is spacing out looking at his or her truck outside. And that's the most fun, because I can compare things. I can see, oh what was he doing? What is he trying to get them to do? If I do it myself, I might feel it, but I can't see myself that well.

Jonathan Shear's perception of auras is reminiscent of driving on the roadways in the summer. "It's like the air is just a little bit different." However, around martial arts masters and yogis, he used to see them really clearly. He recalls tournaments in which a high level teacher would "take a line up." Moving through a line of black belts, one after another, Shear realized that he'd see golden balls around the true masters. Other times, when working out with someone, he'd feel himself go "OOOOP" and find himself inside his partner's ball of energy. Years later, Jonathan is more removed from martial arts and the visual auras are not as prominent.

I just see a bit on people now. Just a little, except around somebody like Maharishi. Actually, just standing there; he would play with my mind the way no one has ever done to me. I have a strong, stubborn mind, but he would play with it the way my judo master would play with my body.

Carole's newfound ability to see her own aura through *ichuan* standing revealed to her an incredible blue.

It is just shockingly beautiful blue. And I have had more experiences meditating where I actually feel myself filled with energy. Not a color so much as transparency. It's kind

120

of hard to explain, but I had a really amazing experience just a few nights ago when I just—it really felt like you could see through me, but I still had a really pearly sensation. I knew where my boundaries were, but it was real pearly, not even so much something to see, but the sensation. But if I was standing outside myself, I could see right through me except for that glimmer.

Carole is also known to see spirits just as she is falling asleep.

I see people moving—all kinds of people—really, really, clearly. It's not like large people, but glimmers of them, and they sort of move through and do different things. Some of them are angry, some of them are sad, some are young, some are old. It's just really a wonder, kind of lying back and letting them move about.

Lynn often experiences what she calls "visual oddness," which includes not just colors, but seeing things where there's not really something there, and other perceptions of energy. The phenomenon happens frequently when she practices on her own, although the intensity grows within a group. One time in a qigong class, she says, a mirage started splitting itself away from her teacher so that by the end of the set there were two of him.

There was the real him and then there was the other one, which sort of got built with his center being the last thing that was filled in. Part of me was just sort of watching this and hoping it didn't stop, you know? This probably has something to do with my being cross eyed, but as he was being built and filled in, Carole's face [Carole was standing in the front row] was in the center of him. I could sort of see her face with his hollow body all around.

At another class, with a different teacher,

We would step right, but imagine as hard as we could, we were stepping left. Then step left, imagine as hard as

121

you could that you were stepping right. And forward and back also. And so you actually take a physical step forward first, but you imagine while you're doing it, you're taking a step back. When you get into it for a while, you sort of feel that meditation feeling like you're all around outside your body—separate from your body. David said to me after class that he saw my aura stepping the way I wasn't. And I swear I saw that on him, too.

After years of reflection on these regular supersensory episodes, Lynn says, "What it's doing is making me more open to other people and more accepting of other people." In other words, there is a breakdown of barriers, between a person and their energy field, and Lynn's sensors that can now take in those higher vibrations whether they are self-generated or generated by another. That opening includes a release of emotional barriers.

Auras, as we saw with Chenoa and Maria, can also be felt. The emotional state translates into an energy field that we pick up through various senses. For example, my son saw my anger as brown. Chenoa can feel energy fields more strongly than she can see them, and Maria was experiencing others' emotional states. That intermingling of energies in a setting where it gains coherence is of great inspiration to Maggie Newman.

The other day we had a class of only five people. It was a class that had been studying for a long time, and they had the usual: each person has a different personality, the things that they will do that get in the way, which will be the same as they always do. But then, we suddenly somehow got into something that was very deep, but it started from each individual having something to work on. After a while, it captured my interest because I saw five people begin to look more and more like full human beings, and more and more they stayed together as a group. To me, that's the ideal thing. Most people think they have to do one or the other. They either stay with everybody else or they do their own thing for it. The class was willing to try to stick together…

Their faces become more comfortable; their bodies become more comfortable. At the same time, they're sticking more and more with each other. So it was an expression of what I think is possible, but there were just five people in class. Sometimes if you have a large class, there are too many waves going in different directions. This was more interesting for me to watch than the usual bumping and struggling, or treating staying together as if it's a chore and as if one has to give up something to do that. So I actually found people doing a better form than I'd seen them do in a long time— more full form. And more relaxed individuals – they all looked like individuals. They don't look like the Rockettes, they look like they're fully themselves—comfortable in changing when everybody else changes. That's the point. You've got to be willing to change.

Carolyn became more sensitive to everything around her, including objects.

I like secondhand things—things that have had a previous owner. I feel very attracted to the energy in objects that I've had or are before me—things that are either secondhand or antiques. I feel a big part of my selection process is a subjective call of the energy. Certain things have a heaviness to them—but not a bad heaviness—just kind of a nice substantial drink to them that feels good to me.

Clairvoyance is another paradigm by which one knows the essence of energies. In Leyla's medical qigong work, her primary mode of sensing is "knowingness."

I'm just drawn to a particular area. … I've learned to sense energetic cores and between them, or dredge the qi and stuff like that, but mostly I'm just drawn to particular areas. I'll spend more time. I'll decide to work on the head area more, because I see it feels good.

Stephen Watson, a world champion push hands player, teacher, and healer, explains:

> I don't experience it as my sense of touch is better, my sense of taste is different than most people's … it may be, but I only know about mine. … But my experience is that those extrasensory perceptions are extrasensory. They don't have to do with my vision or my hearing, or my feeling. It's like they directly enter my body mind. … When I try to describe them, I might describe them visually or in terms of the auditory experience or something, but that's just looking for a way to share the experience.

Mystical or supersensory experience was much more common in earlier times, when taiji practice required an intense apprenticeship with a master, oftentimes to the exclusion of day work. Echoing the *Nei-yei* which advises holding the numinous mind within, and not letting the senses disturb it (Roth, 1999, p. 68), the thirteenth-century anthology *The Book of Harmony and Balance*, Ancestor Lü reminds us very clearly that expanded perceptions of the senses are not the endgame of the practice.

> Stabilizing the Body
> The sublime principle of Complete Reality
> Is not hard to practice;
> Just avoid pursuing things,
> Chasing sound and form.
> When illusions do not invade you,
> Feelings naturally end;
> When the unified mind is unaffected,
> How can thoughts arise?
> Get rid of discrimination of others and self,
> Preserve the celestial design;
> Take yin and yang in hand,
> Join tranquility and development.

I tell the eminent people
Who cultivate the elixir,
When you don't indulge in the senses,
The essence is complete and clear.
—Ancestor Lü (Cleary, 1999, p. 346)

Psychic Children

The difference between the ordinary middle aged player who discovers a new world of frequency and those who have always been open to psychic information is wide. For child-psychics turned adult, taiji creates a path to ground oneself in the world without closing off the stream. For some, such as Tom M., it reopened a conduit he had closed off in childhood. Others find the practice provides a different set of techniques with which to work with information—information that appears far more detailed than it does for nonprodigies. Regardless, the vividness of their experiences are a beacon to those just glimpsing their own potential as spiritual beings through extrasensory perception, or those who discover quite by accident that their "very sensitive" children actually have psychic abilities. Master martial artists are particularly appreciative of their psychic abilities, as precognition and extrasensory perception release them from the constraints of time in assessing and responding to a situation and also provide extra insight about an opponent. An aura, for example, can reveal illness or structural weakness. Or, that flash of insight could be the gift of the half second needed to anticipate and neutralize a strike.

A young Micaela did not realize that other kids weren't playing with balls of energy at lunchtime until she was twelve. Even so, she did get a couple of friends to play a gentle game of diaphanous catch with her. Prone to precognition, she walked home every day from school thinking, "I'd really like to see that episode of the Simpsons tonight." She was regularly rewarded. Similarly, she tends to pick up on other people's thoughts easily saying words at the same time. (Jinx!)

Sarah describes struggling with psychic information her entire life, especially handling conflict with her brothers who hated her knowing their secrets. But she also recognizes that she uses it to compensate for her listening deficiencies. "My hearing is kind of dyslexic. The sounds go in and get jumbled up and don't get sorted out. When I'm tired, I can't hear very well, so I'll rely a lot on energetics and just what I perceive."

Lee, who is also a reiki healer, comes from a family of highly sensitive individuals, so her psychic tendencies were never questioned as a child. In fact, when an episode materialized she was usually invited to talk about it. Her clairvoyant events were frequent and wide ranging and included precognition, empathy, auras, out of body experiences, etc. She heard things before they were spoken and knew things before they happened. Lee also just knew things about other people. As a precursor to her taiji study, she discovered at the wee age of seven that she could move without moving, and she tested her abilities. Despite the acceptance of her family, she was told, "People are going to think that's odd if you do that." Or, "people aren't going to believe you."

It's interesting because it almost sounds like make believe. But you know there are certain sensations that go on with energy that you become aware of…or the sense that something's hurt, you are drawn to it.

This was a part of play for Lee. From picking up rocks to gardening by feeling at her grandma's side, Lee learned to talk to the plants to learn where they would be happy. That back and forth exploration of energy was how she experienced the world.

Not surprisingly, Lee is a natural healer, and she is drawn not only to people who are hurt, but where they hurt.

If your hand's on it or if you follow the inner voice, or you follow without question, energy will lead you to many different things. Everything has a different feeling energy. I knew early on that I could see life force energy around different things—plants, or people or animals—whatever.

126

... You get these urges that you follow. Energy patterns can be anything from thought to heat. It's almost empathic. It's a sensory thing. So I was just always aware—and aware of people's feelings.

As a college student, Lee studied sociology and has worked in social services and human resources. Working with groups and people with special needs, Lee was trained to watch body language for information. What her professors probably would not have predicted is that in this setting, Lee's psychic ability manifested itself through out of body experiences.

If I was thinking about the other person, I would all of a sudden find myself looking across at myself from basically the position they were in, or from their eyes...or [from] an aerial view. So you're there in the body, but then again, all of a sudden you're somewhere else—but you come back.

As a teenager, Lee tested her ability trying to understand it better. For example, she'd ask herself if she knew what that person was going to do before they did it? Or was it that her thoughts controlled what happened?

Through different phases of my life, sometimes I chose not to listen. And when I chose not to listen or respond to a feeling or an urge or a message—being willful —something always got screwed up. And, you know, I knew.

Coming to taiji later in life, Lee notes that when she does reiki she feels energy in the heart whereas in taiji, it is centered in the dantien. Stephe was also a psychic child.

It's more a question of when I realized that that wasn't what everybody had, or everybody could speak about, or everybody was in tune with. So, for me, it didn't feel like a change to become aware of these energies, although I have to say the ones that register in my memory's bookmarks were distressing energetics. You know, prickly feelings and undertones in people's expressions—that sort of thing. And so those stuck in my mind. My first idea of answering the question, "Wow, I used to be more attuned to the bad vibes, but I think that's not true. It's just those are the ones that register and stay with you. ... The only change that I had ... was when I first got glasses, I remember putting them on and saying, "I didn't realize there was that experience of the world to be had." I had never seen it. I didn't have the eyeglass experience with energetics where now I'm awake to this whole other world.

Practice of the internal arts helped Stephe learn to trust his ability and expand the amplitude of those energetics.

In other words, those experiences can be louder to me, and they can affect more than a small part of me. When you change the size of the wave, what it affects is different. So a long bass wave doesn't affect a small thing. Because it bypasses it. And so by adjusting the amplitude up or down, it actually can affect more of me. But I don't think the scope of the vision—I'll say 'vision' but it's not visual—the scope of the experience, that vision, isn't any different. But my trust in it is.

Linda, like her mother, grew up dreaming, or hearing, messages she needed to hear, particularly if one of her many siblings was in trouble. She likens the transmission to being in a waking dream.

Now, I feel like if I want to know, I can actually reach out. One of my brothers has been in detention for a year because of drugs. In the old days I would say, "Well, I haven't dreamed anything, I know he's okay." Now I feel like when I go reach out, and I feel him, I know whether or not he's alive.

The common thread among these qi savants is that taiji helped them frame their perceptions, ground the energy, and find communities of people who were having similar energetic experiences.

Creativity and Artists

> *The Clairvoyant Reality does not have discrete or separate entities in it; attempts at describing experiences and perceptions in it are bound to fail. The physicist has his mathematics, which he can use to describe and manipulate concepts in the Clairvoyant Reality. Perhaps the most successful modes of expression for experiences in this reality are music and nonrepresentational art. When we listen to Haydn's The Creation or the Brandenburg Concertos or respond to a Klee, a Miró, or certain Picassos, we are likely to get a strong sense of much that the mystic is talking about.*
>
> —Lawrence LeShan (LeShan, 2003, p. 74)

Taiji practitioners strive for *wuji*, the infinite. That shift into sciousness, open to flow and free of mind state obstacles, is familiar to artists, writers, and musicians. The consensus is that their taiji practice helps them and has great impact on them as artists. That feeling of *wu wei*, action without doing, is familiar, and the practice provides a set of tools to find that place more readily and regularly.

As Jonathan Shear pointed out, any practice that becomes refined enough, no matter how mundane—from shining shoes to painting barn walls—can become a technique to transcend just as *Zuangzi*'s legendary Daoist butcher demonstrated[8]. The effort that one makes in doing a repetitive activity becomes so small that it just starts

---

[8] Cook Ding was cutting up an ox for Lord Wenhui. At every touch of his hand, every heave of his shoulder, every move of his feet, every thrust of his knee—zip! zoop! He slithered the knife along with a zing, and all was in perfect rhythm, as though he were performing the dance of the Mulberry Grove or keeping time to the Jingshou music.

happening. The ordinary person might get really bored by it. The person who knows something about enlightenment, keeps doing it until it becomes a technique from which to transcend into a shifted state of consciousness.

In practical terms, photographer and cinematographer Ken Van Sickle explains that the taiji practice allows your left brain to relax and lets the subconscious respond more through the right brain. That right brain presence, he says, is the key to differentiating between craft and art.

"Ah, this is marvelous!" said Lord Wenhui. "Imagine skill reaching such heights!"

Cook Ding laid down his knife and replied, "What I care about is the Way, which goes beyond skill. When I first began cutting up oxen, all I could see was the ox itself. After three years I no longer saw the whole ox. And now—now I go at it by spirit and don't look with my eyes. Perception and understanding have come to a stop and spirit moves where it wants. I go along with the natural makeup, strike in the big hollows, guide the knife through the big openings, and follow things as they are. So I never touch the smallest ligament or tendon, much less a main joint.

"A good cook changes his knife once a year—because he hacks. I've had this knife of mine for nineteen years and I've cut up thousands of oxen with it, and yet the blade is as good as though it had just come from the grindstone. There are spaces between the joints, and the blade of the knife has really no thickness. If you insert what has no thickness into such spaces, then there's plenty of room—more than enough for the blade to play about in. That's why after nineteen years the blade of my knife is still as good as when it first came from the grindstone.

"However, whenever I come to a complicated place, I size up the difficulties, tell myself to watch out and be careful, keep my eyes on what I'm doing, work very slowly, and move the knife with the greatest subtlety, until flop! the whole thing comes apart like a clod of earth crumbling to the ground. I stand there holding the knife and look all around me, completely satisfied and reluctant to move on, and then I wipe off the knife and put it away."

"Excellent!" said Lord Wenhui. "I have heard the words of Cook Ding and learned how to care for life!" —Zhuangzi (Watson, 2003, pp. 45–7)

If that's not happening, then you're not really doing the art. I mean two thirds of what you're doing is subconscious. And if you haven't tapped that, what you're doing is your using your muscles. That creates nice paintings or nice literature, but it's not art. It can't be. You have to be tapping into that.

Furthermore, "Every art by definition contributes to every other art," says Ken. Remembering Cheng Man Ching who was a master of five arts—taiji, medicine, calligraphy, poetry, and painting—each one of them made him more of an artist in every other one. "Each art has its own specific rules and principles and concepts, and each one has something in common with another art as well as something that is different. Each difference contributes to the parallel universe of the other art."

David Hawkins describes the creative process as tapping into higher harmonics:

What the genius arrives at is a new harmonic. Every advance in human consciousness has come through a leap from a lower attractor pattern ot its higher harmonic. Posing the original question activates an attractor; the answer lies within its harmonic.

... Genius and creativity, then, are subjectively experienced as a *witnessing*; it's a phenomenon that bypasses the individual self or ego. The capacity to finesse genius can be learned—though often only through painful surrender—when the phoenix of genius arises out of the ashes of despair after a fruitless struggle with the unsolvable. Out of defeat comes victory; out of failure, success; and out of humbling, true self-esteem. (Hawkins, 2002, pp. 196–98)

To Ken, the early contributions of taiji to his work in film was an outgrowth of the physical training. As a gaffer and a grip, he discovered the influence of push hands in his sensitivity while pushing a dolly. When he moved onto handheld camera work, he could hold the camera and move it around as if it were part of his body.

What I continue to develop, and it continues much because of taiji, is the ability to change the way things look to me. It's not an aura or anything. It's just all of a sudden I look. I see that I'm on this planet. And I see it as that. I'm this visitor on this planet. I see it differently. It just goes into a different look. And I really like that. It's a wonderful planet. It's got trees and clouds and beautiful things. And I like looking at it from some place else. I can see it as differently as—Oh, I know that that's a maple tree and this is cement and this is a rubber thing for kids, but I just see it as what it is. Purely.

Linda describes a similar perspective when writing. After five years of work, she discovered that a ritual of meditation and slow movement were key to getting the last 50,000 words of a novel written. "The words would just come out." Asked to describe the change in consciousness that accompanies this state of flow, she says, "It feels like I'm physically leaning back into something. Then I'm very aware of everything around me and being outside myself—outside of my skin."

Lynn also feels herself move in and out of this state of sciousness. "Sometimes I'm painting, and all of a sudden it's like somebody else did it. Somebody else painted that piece. The style is more impressionistic. I would say it is more a suggestion of what the thing is, but it's so perfect that I leave it alone." Taiji training also has influenced her composition, with the path the eye is directed to follow becoming more and more spiraled.

In addition to a lifetime in martial arts, Eli also plays congas. "When you let yourself go, *it* comes out of your palms." The sense of freedom is accompanied by a natural shift into a trance state. "When we were kids we used to close our eyes and just play. It wasn't coordinated or anything. We'd just keep playing. The next thing you knew everybody was in tune."

Tom D. credits his capacity to sustain a career as a writer to taiji because it gave him a framework for his craft.

I was very fortunate. At one point, toward the end of his time in America with us, Professor [Cheng Man Ching] taught a beginner's brush class. All we ever did was lines across and down the page with watery ink on newspaper because we weren't able to get past the inability to make straight lines without sloshing around. And, he began the class by saying to do the brush was fairly simple. You put those … and he sort of gestured … He said you put both feet flat in the ground, you sit up straight, you move from your center, you use both your arms and you go like this. He said, "For me, this is like taiji. It's another form of meditation."

And, in the moment that he said that, I realized that all of my conflicts about ambition and accomplishment and having an audience to appreciate my work, and all these other sort of outwardly facing things that artists become artists to achieve on some level—well they just evaporated for me. I came to understand that just like taiji, you are a taiji person if you do taiji. It's not like getting a grade or being good or bad at it. You do it or you don't do it, but that's all there is. Someone's a writer if they write. But it is irrelevant to who you are, and that liberated me to pursue different kinds of writing in my life, to pursue different kinds of art with a kind of freedom and confidence and also with an essential centeredness that I'd never have achieved otherwise. And it was in that single moment that my whole life as a writer was transformed.

Libby also cannot give enough credit to her taiji training in her development as a musician. She says it took her farther than she ever could have gone with just her musical training. Starting with the practical approach of grounding, she abandoned her penchant for high heels, put her feet on the ground, and developed a sense of body awareness. In addition to helping with technique, that also helped her physical and mental equipoise. Integrating the martial attitude of taiji training was also important to her success.

Playing music, there is a degree to which you're out there as a warrior. And sometimes it might be something as basic as just simply having concentration. Having good concentration, being able to ward off the thoughts that come in your head that are random, or the self-doubt, or whatever that might be.

Some of this is as direct as sitting next to somebody that you know wants you to screw up, and at the time I was in those kinds of circles. [I was] able to sit there and play my best, and not lose a lot of energy to deal with those kinds of onslaughts.

... So it is the martial aspect of being centered. It's also the sense of rootedness and concentration. In pretty much all my endeavors that was my limitation. Everybody has strengths and weaknesses, and there is something in their character that is tending towards a weakness. In my case, certainly at the time, it was that I had a very fast, flighty kind of brain. It was hard to just be rooted and sit with something.

Libby also describes a period of time later in her development when all she wanted to practice was long tones. She played them for hours as a kind of meditation and neglected practicing technique or her parts for gigs. "I got a little worried that I would go to gigs and concerts, and I might not be able to actually play the parts. In fact, I played better."

Another principle her taiji teacher talked about was investing in loss. For a Westerner, says Libby, that doesn't mean a thing.

I translated that to "Don't overly invest in winning. Don't overly invest in being on top all the time, don't overly invest in being in control all the time. And I found that what that did for me, opening up the vulnerability, opening up the softness, my own softness—was extremely helpful in terms of receptivity towards music—but also towards other human beings, and even animals ... and in so doing, becoming much stronger.

Libby sees a direct parallel to the way one opens up through taiji and through music. In taiji, every move starts with a neutralization. Martially that means allowing one's opponent to move you and come close. You have to surrender your ego, give up the struggle and trust your technique. Likewise, you can only understand the depth of music if you allow yourself to give yourself up to it, she says. "That is a very similar model in terms of spirituality. The taiji spirituality is imminent. It's in your body. It's in the ground. It's in the grass."

Finding the Inner Shaman

The mystery of natural law is learned from a teacher, but it is based on the celestial order, which circulates throughout the earth. Once the Great Way is accomplished, then miracles, at the extreme end of natural law, are manifested at will, and supernatural powers are unfathomable. Then the sky and earth are like a pouch, sun and moon are in a pot, the minuscule is gigantic, the macrocosm is minute; you can manipulate the cosmos at will, looking upon the universe as a mote of dust. Now integrating, now vanishing, now detached, now present, you enter the hidden and emerge in the evident; space itself disappears. You can even employ spirits and ghosts and make thunder and lightning.

—Ancestor Lü (Cleary, 2000, p. 109)

As discussed before, the disintegration of barriers and softening of the edges between subject and object that the taiji player notices through sensual stimuli extend one's range of perception, moving one's consciousness into the realms of the mystical, or paranormal, and atuning everyday consciousness to greater and greater awareness of extended frequency. As William James puts it,

[S]tates of mystical intuition may be only very sudden and great extensions of the ordinary "field of consciousness." ... the extension itself would ... consist in an immense spreading of the margin of the field, so that knowledge ordinarily transmarginal would become included, and the ordinary margin would grow more central (James, 1910).

As taiji players enter these higher levels of consciousness, many of their accounts take on shamanistic shadings. Loosely defined, shamanism is a practice of indigenous cultures that connects the human to the spirit world. Interconnectedness is a central tenet. Practices vary around the world, from inducing trance via hallucinogens, sensory

136

deprivation, kinetic activity, and meditation, but most accounts describe attunement with nature and interaction with vivid, culturally influenced spirit imagery (Kalweit, 1988, p. 124).

In Daoist lore, the wanderings of the sages, their return to nature, and purity of thought hold the preagricultural societies of paleolithic and mesolithic man as an ideal. Their example of living outside political and social structures is encouraged in the earliest texts from the third century BCE and show man attuned to the universe in ways that both attend to their physical needs for food and shelter but are also anchored in mystical awareness (Kohn, 2017, p. 65). It has been theorized that the phenomenon of changed states of consciousness was discovered as ancient hunters stood in stillness awaiting prey. Those standing meditative postures were recorded in cave paintings, petroglyphs and art in cultures around the world, hinting at the esteem with which they were held (Cohen, 1997, pp. 133–6).

Living on the fringes of society in close relationship with nature, Daoist shamans gave birth to many of the ideas that taiji revolves around. The fundamental Daoist cosmology, according to Laozi, starts with One (Dao) which blossoms into the duality of yin and yang and opens to the myriad things. That includes the five elements and the ancient symbolic animals integral to the Daoist arts in general, including taiji forms, qigong, astrology, divination, feng shui, and acupuncture. The process of both the sage and taiji practitioner is to ease back down this chain of creativity, returning to the embrace of source energy.

> Many of their powers are similar to the abilities of shamans. Daoist immortals heal the sick, exorcise demons or beasts, make rain or stop it, foretell the future, prevent disasters, call upon wild animals as helpers, and remain unharmed by water and fire, heat and cold. Control over the body, a subtle harmony with the forces of nature, as well as an easy relationship with gods and spirits, ghosts and demons are equally characteristic of successful shamans as of the immortals of the Dao (Kohn, 2012, pp. 7–8).

In modern times—moving away from the cacophony of electronic frequency, combustion engines, and inorganic environments—the taiji player, outdoors, relaxes into his structure (the principle of *song*) and connects his body to heaven and earth—attuned to the frequencies of water, earth, rocks, and trees, allowing the Schumann Resonance to ring more brightly through his vessel. While in this altered state of consciousness, one can enter into different relationships with animals and the environs.

> In reality, there are principles of chemistry, physics, and biology involved here. Extending the principle, if people pay attention to the minute and subtle changes inside the body while sitting cross-legged, this enables people to sense the subtle changes in vibration frequencies on the surface of the earth. Equilibrium exercise, standing with your back to a tree bathing in its energy, is seeking to assimilate your "field" to the "field" of the tree; if small animals also actually practice cultivation in the presence of humans, that means that they too are tuning their energy field (Kaiguo and Shunchao, 1996, p. 197).

"The shaman keeps the human discourse from rigidifying," writes David Abram in *The Spell of the Sensuous*, "and keeps the perceptual membrane fluid and porous, ensuring the greatest possible attunement between the human community and the animate earth, between the familiar and the fathomless" (Abram, 1996, p. 256).

Sedona, Arizona is known for its intense natural energies and indigenous spiritual history. Now also a center for psychic new agers, Sedona's power emerges from the red rock vortices (spiraling centers of energy arising from or descending into the earth). For many, those spiraling electromagnetics have the effect of amplifying frequencies and changing states of consciousness[9].

---

[9] Master Wang Liping maps not only apertures of the body to planets in the universe, but also longitudinal and latitudinal lines to the meridians and apertures of the body. In fact, Liping notes that the naval gate of life corresponds to the oil

Scheila's first trip to Sedona to attend a taiji workshop unexpectedly turned into a shamanistic event starting with a hike to what is known as the Shaman's Cave. She had never before done any Native American shamanic work but found herself drawn to sit by a painted white horse on the wall. Suddenly,

> I did this falcon thing. I don't know how to describe it other than I could feel my feathers. And you know how a bird sits on a branch or something with its wings at its side. That's how I could feel. I could feel all of that. There's the depressions in the floor of the cave. Somehow, instinctively I knew where to sit, where I had sat in the past and that those impressions were for grinding colors—ochre—for sacred work.

Later that weekend, with several others on a back road, a falcon flew parallel to the van. Highly attuned at this point, Scheila pointed it out, and the driver stopped the van so they could get out to watch. Scheila recalls the falcon putting on a little show, flying in a taiji-like spiraling figure eight pattern.

While on her annual hike to Sedona's Bell Rock, Carolyn saw tiny white flowers growing close to the ground.

> I was aware of this little bunch of voices—like little children laughing, giggling and saying, "Hi, hi." It was like the flowers had this little voice. They were all giving out this greeting to us as we were walking through in a very innocent, cheerful, playful way ...
>
> I wasn't physically hearing it. It wasn't reverberating in my ear, but I was very aware of it. Those little flowers had this presence—a spirit—that was attempting to communicate.

On another visit, Carolyn was overcome by the urge to lie down

---

fields of the Middle East while its opposite point, the Gate of Death in the small of the back, corresponds to the Bermuda Triangle (Kaiguo and Shunchao, 1996).

in a riverbed. She had been having a touchy year and was feeling pretty miserable. But in that safe haven, she cried, released grief, and talked to her deceased grandfather. The following year, walking through that same area with a group, her companions seemed to be aware of her grandfather's residual energy, including the soft quality of his voice and the things he was saying. "That was strange, surreal, somewhat paranormal, but nevertheless, there it is. I can't prove it. It's just what I experienced," recalls Carolyn.

Another participant in those annual Tai Chi Alchemy weekends in Sedona was Stephe Watson. The group hikes and explores the energies around Cathedral and Bell rocks, and on Stephe's first trip to Bell Rock he was at first taken by the irresistible urge to climb higher and higher. But, as he reached the shoulders of the formation, he found himself weak and deflated.

Not in my legs or in my cardio—I want to say the wind went out of my sails, but it was the want that went out of my sails. So, inevitably, I collapse into a sobbing pile of forlorn. Which leads to crying for other things ... people you miss, or experiences you miss, or both miss in terms of your past and you don't have them, and also miss as in the arrow that didn't hit its mark.

Anyway, this crying continued for two days, two and half days. Either crying already, or crying at the drop of a hat. Essentially being reduced to a formless heap. And a shuddering kind of crying. I'd already understood yin as a release. And of course that release is with the body. Sink in your legs. Sink in your root. Drop your shoulders; let your tailbone sink. All this. Release. And I also understood it in terms of intellectual release, release from expectations. Release from your standard sensory apparatus and so forth. So intellectually I understood that it was emotional release. But I hadn't done that. Certainly not this extremely, anyway. And I know that the mind and the heart are the same thing, but I had been practicing the release with the mind and the body. And so it was almost like my experience wasn't so much being on Bell Rock but being in the face of the awe, which is an overused word, but the awe—of yin.

The next year, Stephe recalls being drawn to a smaller butte between Bell and Cathedral rocks.

All of a sudden I was running. My eyes were closed. I just ran, ran, ran. I must have stayed on the path because I didn't stumble or run into a bush, and at one point I stopped. A snake went from left to right, through my legs, from off the path, through my legs, around the path and off the path. I was about to access the standard part of me, which is to analyze, comment, observe, basically make ready for memory of that experience. Then I started running. I don't know why I was running. And I was certainly running faster, it felt, than I could run for my weight and age. I only stopped for four seconds or something for the snake. It wove like a yin yang ...

I got up to this little butte. I clambered up. From the top I could see the rest of our group way at the beginning of the path kind of starting to spider out on their particular paths. I was already at the top. I stripped off all my clothes and was practicing the earth element of xingyi. It was just bad practice. ... closing the hands wrong and getting the hand under when it should be over. ... it had this fervor—this furious or passionate element to it that it hadn't ever had because I'm trained not to do that...

The revelation finally rose to my awareness. I thought "the rock, through the earth, through that phase, through that state, through that element: I understand gravity.

Sensing that the lesson was not over, he later taught a short segment on it knowing that teaching others is often a means to synthesize our own understanding. The realization that Stephe was able to give words to is that

Gravity is just the earth's looking for community, so it draws things in just the way that we do. But, of course, we do it by making ourselves consciously fit in. But the earth doesn't need your consciousness. And it doesn't need to change what it is. It just is itself.

Synchronicity subsequently reinforced the lesson for Stephe. The next day a friend who had taken a picture of him on the butte from afar asked if he could use the image in a calendar he was producing. He wanted that photo to represent the gravity month. That another could tune into gravity through the image was a renewal of trust for Stephe.

Power is still, affirms David Hawkins. "It's like a standing field that doesn't move. Gravity itself, for instance, doesn't move against anything. Its power moves all objects within its field" (Hawkins, 2002). The shaman taps into that power as does the deep rooted taiji player.

Beyond the obvious parallel emphases on nature and animal qualities, gaining power for healing, and their use in conflict, taiji and shamanism also share a focus on changes in consciousness. Shamans' accounts from across cultures feature striking tales as journeyers take leave of their bodies and enter into worlds of spirits and animals. Acknowledging the historical connection, taiji, too, affects changes in consciousness says Don Miller, who after working extensively with a man named Medicine Singer, came to see the practices as almost synonymous.

There's no single taiji state. But taiji enables and facilitates exploring a variety of body mind states other than the one you're normally tripping around with—tripping as in tripping over things, stumbling around. And, there's not just one; there are many, and in fact, each of the major postures and associated *jings* or qualities in the taiji form, such as *peng, lu, ji, an*, etc… are actually complete altered states. They're completely different states of mind, body, spirit, perception, vision. Different parts of the brain are being used. You see differently. Your body functions differently. In other words, this idea of doing the form with a consistent quality throughout is actually only one way of doing taiji, and it's not really the most interesting. It's useful for meditation because you don't have to go through all these changes. But actually, the form, as I'm now understanding it, is a journey through a whole series of different states of body and mind. The consciousness that you inhabit when you're doing press is completely different than the consciousness you inhabit when you do rollback. Until you understand that, you're missing out on three quarters of what there is in taiji.

So, my understanding of taiji now is that it's very shamanistic. You go into different states of being through certain psychophysical practices, and you come back with the boon, or the benefit, of that journey which you then integrate into the rest of yourself and your life.

Unless you do extreme taiji practices, and there are plenty, the journeys are short. They may only be a minute. Or they may only be 10 seconds. But they are definitely journeys into other states than the so-called normal state.

It is not only people who undergo changes in consciousness doing taiji forms. Ken Van Sickle notes that many people who do the taiji form out in nature witness animals act differently, too.

Even people who don't do it that well will see the animals being less afraid of them. In fact, once, I was on a porch of a house near Woodstock, New York and a swallow landed on my arm. I was doing ward off, [also known as Grasp Sparrow's Tail] the swallow landed right on my ward off and facing me, just looking me in the eyes. I stopped doing the form, but, with taiji movement, I walked over to the window and I knocked on the window with my right hand and my two friends were inside and looked outside and saw the swallow sitting there; they were very surprised. I walked back in repulse monkey, and [as] I started to do the next movement it flew away.

Lynn often practices out in the farm fields on the Connecticut River flood plains where she walks her dog, Nikki. Normally, as soon as she sees a hawk, it's gone. However, if she is doing taiji, she says, they will watch her. In return, she can look at them, and they don't fly away.

Lynn's pets also have predictable reactions to certain energies as she practices. Her cat, with certain moves, will grab Lynn's ankle. "She'll wrap herself around my feet and kind of hold on. It makes her kind of feisty, but still want to be close." Other times the cat curls her front feet under her and just purrs with half closed eyes.

Lynn's dog, Nikki, is particularly dramatic during xingyi. "It can make her crazy. She'll get that sort of worried 'Do you still love me?' kind of look and attitude."

Both animals get underfoot when Lynn practices a bagua circle walk. "The weird thing is, is they lie down at the point where I usually start my circle. They won't do it as I'm starting, but after I've been going around for a while, they'll lie down in the spot where I started."

Nikki also is drawn to push hands. Several times during push hands practice, intent on exploring subtle energies, Lynn would stop to discover Nikki sitting right in the middle of the circle between her feet and her partner's feet. She then spent the remainder of the evening in a mellowed out qi trance rather than in her usual perky, playful state.

A year or so into his study, Bob went on a fishing trip to the Florida Keys with a friend. They stayed on a beautiful spot of land between the Gulf of Mexico and the Atlantic Ocean. One morning, with the tides moving softly, Bob started his form.

> It was one of those really deep practices you get when you were first learning that suddenly surprise you. As I turned doing Fair Lady at the Shuttles, there were three blue herons and four egrets sitting in a semicircle watching me. ... And when I finished, they left.

In their account of the modern master, Wang Liping, Chen Kaiguo and Zheng Shunchao explain that opening the third eye makes one

144

"capable of inner vision and thus can successfully cultivate refinement in conjunction with the cycles of the sun and moon. This is followed by 'external radiation of internal energy,' which can draw small animals to you" (Kaiguo and Shunchao, 1996, p. 30).

David Chandler, part Cherokee, is a pipe carrier in that tradition and has many stories of being attuned to nature through taiji. The animal frolics are particularly poignant to him because they are the earliest practices of taiji and are directly connected to the ancients who taught people how to survive. "Some qigong practices go back to when people were in caves," says David. "The ones who sat still all the time during the deep winter, preserved some of their energy, but they weren't strong enough to live." Those who exercised survived.

David also notes the prehistoric journey of peoples from Asia to America, carrying with them the shamanistic traditions that they practiced in China. For example, the Diné (as the Navaho refer to themselves) mandala symbol is nearly identical to the yin yang symbol. The white and black fishes within an s-shaped circle, albeit without the dot, represent night and day and polarities of the universe. That symbolic connection, says David, goes back to primordial times. "So for me, what my witness is around, is that taijiquan is a type of shamanic dance, if you will. It is a way of accessing the deep layers of consciousness of human beings."

This came alive several years ago when David was filming the five animal frolics in Montana just south of Yellowstone. The first shot was the tiger frolic. Seeing a great, big boulder out in the middle of the field that must have been left by a glacier, David thought this would be the perfect place for tigers. While his crew was getting set up, he walked around the boulder. First he saw a big hole underneath it. Then he saw the claw marks and the grass lifting up as if something had just been there. Realizing there was a mountain lion, his body shrunk in reaction. Before having time to think he heard, "Action." Trained to that command, he immediately composed himself and thought, "'Okay, it went away, it must be full. I'm okay, I'm going to be safe; I'm going to be a good cat right now. Just another big cat.' And so I occupied that mind place and finished the shot."

The next animal they filmed was the bear. As David was getting ready, he looked over and saw a tree that had the markings of where a bear had stripped the bark. He then looked around and saw bear prints.

Next they were setting up to do the crane movement, and a group of Sand Hill Cranes flew by. David's thought at these extraordinary synchronistic displays was "It's just tuning into the consciousness of nature, and it responds 'here, we're going to supply you with this.'"

As they stopped at their next location to film the dragon movement, David thought. "Now, obviously, where's the dragon going to show up?" Then he looked around and saw snake holes and lizards.

Moving out on a rig to film the final animal—the deer—a herd of them walked by while the crew was working.

> On the way back, the mountain lion actually stalked us. It walked behind us. That was an experience for me about connecting with animals—connecting with nature in the sense of becoming one with it on such a level that you feel that your human aspect reaches its fullest by going back to its deep nature of animal—and to its higher nature of what we will become as well. That higher aspect of what happens when we really tune—it's like that duofold thing in a sense. No ego/full ego. Or [being] completely aware of your animal nature and completely aware of your highest spiritual becoming.

On another occasion, David was demonstrating a five element form in New Mexico. It was right after he'd been on a month long retreat with Chungliang Al Huang of the Living Dao Foundation. As he went through a section named for the wind, describing each movement and how it relates to the wind, a profound attunement set in, not only with David, but also with the spectators.

> When you play taiji, you pay attention to your environment. You connect with it, you merge with it, you are the center of the mandala that looks out around you, and you see the big circle of the sky. And you connect with

146

the sky, you connect with the earth, you connect with the dropping of the leaves, the movement of the insects, the flight of the bird, and in accepting all that and just being with it without judging it, without judging yourself, without having lots of words come up, you just sit in the center of that and let it all happen. And what happens inside you—your heart is moving, you're breathing, and your thoughts are moving naturally too—but you try to let the flow happen and not attach to everything.

At one point he turned to face the audience and with the wind behind him, he pushed. They all bent backwards. The next time he came around the same thing happened, only now their jaws are also dropped in awe and they are asking, "how did he get to control the wind like that?" In reality, David was not miraculously controlling nature, but deeply connecting to it.

When you're in an event like push hands you don't try to control them; you control yourself. And you become the wind. You become the water; you become the fire. You become the metal, and in doing that you allow them to tip themselves over. You allow the event to unfold like a ripened fruit falling from a tree on its own accord. It's ready.

For those focusing on a micro level with one aspect of nature, like David with the wind, trees are particularly accessible as their yang aspect broadcasts energy above ground. Jeff, five or six years into his study, was meditating with a tree as part of his push hands class. He'd chosen a tall, skinny, not-too-healthy looking pine tree that was dripping sap. He assumed a rollback posture:

We were supposed to really listen to the partner, i.e. the tree. So I listened in really close, and I got pretty energized and pretty dynamic with the hands, so it wasn't simply listening, it was a listening dynamic—partnering, gonna move sense. At one instant I felt with the tree. "Ah haa, now I've got you." And as soon as that happened, there was almost a crack. I couldn't hear it, but I felt an electric shock kind of thing and was bounced back a couple feet from the tree.

Listening to trees has become a regular event for Jeff, and they sometimes surprise him. Given that it was mid-October and the leaves were falling, a relatively young maple tree showed him that his expectation that there wouldn't be as much energy as usual was false. "I realized there's a lot going on here. It was quite a vibrant day for that tree. I learned that actually it's a very busy time of year for the trees, as they're getting ready for the winter, storing up their energy."

Jeff's sensitivity to trees includes the ability to perceive their individuality, including the distinct feeling of unhappy or sick trees that he describes as having "a sticky kind of energy and almost a sadness coming out." Sometimes this happens when a tree looks healthy on the outside, but also when there are obvious black spots on the leaves or the bark doesn't look healthy.

In Arizona again, Stephe and two companions were hiking at Thumb Butte in Prescott. As they were going down a slope to return to their car, Stephe heard a tree crying. Without analyzing the perception, he walked off the path, down the hill and honed in directly on the crying evergreen that someone had hammered framing nails into. Without thinking he began to yank out nails.

The three inch nails were at about shoulder level, so they should have been difficult to pull out with just his hands, but they weren't.

> I must have gotten three or four nails out when Jim showed up, and he started pulling nails out. A couple of the nails were pretty far overhead so you had to kind of really strain to reach. And, of course, then you don't have leverage, so I remember about half the time we were there was like on the last two nails. And I guess after about 10 minutes we pulled all the nails out—maybe a dozen and a half nails. When we got the last nail out, it stopped crying—which was really an experience that I relate to the word hearing—but I didn't hear the tree making any noise per se. I felt it crying. Then Jim and I both placed our palms on the tree and offered it consoling healing energy.

A beautiful setting one hot August day was the backdrop for Laddie's textbook samadhi experience, in which he experienced a state of complete nondual integration with all around him and dissolution of his sense of self. At the bend of a river, on a beautiful day, he was nearly encircled by the water as he practiced form, qigong and standing as the sun began to set. When finished, he faced West to watch the sunset. The colors were changing and the water reflected the sunlight. Backlight and shadows on the landmarks added to the play of light. Emptied of everyday mind preoccupations from his session, Laddie's perception changed.

> I couldn't give you an amount of time, but I would say three or four minutes where—it wasn't that there was water; it wasn't that there was sunshine; it wasn't that there was shadow; it wasn't that there was me. *It just was.*
>
> I'm a visual person—the only thing about *me* was the eyes that were perceiving. I literally disappeared. And so did everything else in terms of the sun as an object, the water as an object, the structures as an object. Even the place I was standing kind of became something else—shapeless, formless, without material.
>
> And, from somewhere deep inside a critical, judgmental, ego-based aspect of my personality, I took a look at the stillness, the quietness, and the emptiness, and totally rejected it and ran in fear.

Looking back, Laddie recalls that being young and single, with money in his pocket and a lot of free time, he wanted to play, not work at not being. That rejection, which instantaneously came out of nowhere, was a deep, gut reaction to giving up life as it was. To lose duality, explains Laddie, you have to lose an awful lot more. Laddie equates the experience with Biblical references to looking into the face of God and finding it too terrible to behold. Laddie found the abyss by his own efforts without the guidance of a teacher. Lacking preparation, recognition, or any understanding, the experience was overwhelming and frightening, and in a way still haunts him decades later.

I believe in this life once you are given a gift, if you hand it back, you'll fight like hell to ever get it back again. My experience of that is my experience in dealing with addictions. Once you are given the gift of freedom from the addiction, and you decide to pick it up again, you will struggle for a long time in order to regain that freedom. And you know, an addiction is nothing more than a willful abuse of something that you don't need to abuse. It can be any pursuit, but the key word is "willful."

Enlightenment is a damning experience. Because once you are enlightened, you are stuck with it for your lifetime. … And the hard part of this is, if you don't live according to the enlightenment, you will suffer.

Moments of Transcendence

Spontaneous Spiritual Experiences

I am God in a body. Everyone has that feeling, but no one uses it. I do make use of it, and know its results. People think that this feeling is a spiritual trance, but I am not in a trance. I am love. I am in a trance, the trance of love.

—Nijinsky (Acocella, 2007, p. 32)

U nder the surface chatter of these interviews, several people described their taiji experiences to me as "roll your own" satoris and hallucinogenic "unveilings." Pure awe and gratitude for the validation of drug induced revelation are common denominators among these individuals. Their accounts offer no distinguishing features between nondual realization attained through recreational or spiritual use of hallucinogens and those attained through taiji or meditation.

Indeed, Stanislav Grof showed the world that the consciousness journey on the wings of LSD can be achieved far more safely through natural means. His alternative method, Holotropic Breathwork™, and the hallucinogenic experiences they induce, truly are indistinguishable from those induced by drugs (Grof and Bennett, 1993, p. 22). Taiji can also lead people to superconscious states, although not on demand as with drugs or Grof's method.

Many summers ago, as I sat though yet another inane animated movie for kids, finding bright moments watching my giggling son, I watched a psychedelic cartoon portrayal of a bonk on the head with new perspective. Those bold rotating colors harking back to pop art of the sixties still do the trick in cartoons, yet they come out of the familiar experience of altered consciousness. The experience is similar to a pedestrian phenomenon of my own meditations. Enjoyment of the lava lamp-like succession of wild purples, pinks, blue, and mint green really only takes a few moments of concentration on the third eye in a sunny room. That truly is a world of swirling, throbbing, dancing color.

Tim, in his twenties, found taiji through sexual yoga. After ten years of heavy drug and alcohol abuse that started as an adolescent, he turned to martial arts and fully embraced many aspects of Daoist practice, including herbology, diet, and meditation. His desire to be healthy, for himself and for others, was a strong motivation. He also enjoys the power of martial arts.

> Making yourself and another whole again in some way is one of the most incredible feelings in this world. They're two sides of the same coin. You have to learn one to learn the other and to do either well. ... Every amazing experience I've ever had on drugs has been topped by another experience I've had studying Traditional Chinese Medicine.

After Jeff's push hands match with the pine tree that sparkling June morning, he walked down to the beach. It was late morning and the sun was high in the sky. The pebbles and rivulets of water flowing back and forth from the swash of the waves as the tide moved out mesmerized him. The experience was basically the same as when he had experimented with hallucinogenic mushrooms as a teenager on the same beach. He attuned to the elemental flow of water and light from a perch of joyful detachment. "It was gorgeous, and yet it was utterly meaningless at the same time."

On any given day, he says, one can go to the shore and see the pebbles and water. They get thrown by the waves and there is a trail of water that follows the waves back out to sea as the tide recedes.

> In that altered state, physical reality doesn't hitch itself to one's brain. From that state you see the play of elemental energy with sparks and pinpoints of light bouncing off the sun. The motion of the water is highlighted by the

light. It's not that you look at it and say, look at the sun sparkle off the water, isn't it pretty? You see pinprints of energy all around you. It's a detachment from the real, physical thing.

Some forty years ago, Don Miller was driving through Vermont when his thoughts roamed through his activities from the prior weeks. As his mind caromed back and forth, his consciousness started to rise at a very rapid rate.

I knew I was headed within a matter of seconds for cosmic consciousness. I can't tell you exactly what that is, because I didn't go there. But it was some kind of enlightenment, or breakthrough of some kind. However, I also know as I was hurtling upward that if I went there I would get there, but I would not be able to drive the car, the car would crash, and I would die. And it wouldn't matter because I would have obtained cosmic consciousness, but my present incarnation would be over. And I didn't want that. I was not ready for that, and I basically declined the offer.

With an enormous effort of will, I had to sort of pull my sensuousness back into my body, so that I could continue to drive the car. Had I been sitting under a bodi tree or a pine tree, where I was safe, perhaps I would have been able to actually have that breakthrough and still survive physically.

… I wanted to return to those possibilities, but more at the time and place and pace of my choosing rather than just having it happen. So, I've had a lot of wonderful experiences through taiji and since studying taiji, but not exactly a repeat of that one. But I'm not in a rush for it.

Likewise, Luke was driving a truck to South Jersey when he encountered the divine. He worked for an antiques moving company and was carrying a very valuable piece into horse country when he drove into a strong rain and wind storm.

The truck slid into the other lane. There was lightning, and as I pulled [the truck] back into my own lane, I had this experience of everything's [being] lush and green and red and really alive. The horizon went right through my body. Right here at [the] dantien. Down below were roots. So everything from the dantien down was roots, below ground. Everything up here was leaves and branches and rain. It was really strong. It was very visual. Very tactile. These things happen once; they only happen once, but they're lifelong lessons.

A vehement atheist, Jeff was a bit taken aback by his sudden realization that a universal consciousness was part of the game. He has since palpably felt live spirits several times.

There was one time, where I'd just passed through a very difficult time of my life, and I was very grateful to have come through and to be in a happy place. As a lifelong skeptic, atheist, I just spontaneously said, "Thank you, God." There was an immediate answer in a form of an energetic hugging all through my energy field. A very beautiful feeling pulsation throughout the field. [It was a] warmth, throbbing, large, loving energy, which was a real shock to me because there was no God. I said, "Thank you, God." And God said, "Of course. You're welcome. I'm here. I love you"—which blew my socks off. So I go, "really?" and then it came back with the same kind of hug, and of course, just love.

A couple years down the road, at a group meditation, the leader guided the group in bringing light into the body. And she said "Now feel God's appreciation for all that we do." Still a bit skeptical, Jeff dove in.

WHAM it came in. I really felt that compassion ... And it was similar, [but] a little different quality from that other experience. But it was a very powerful experience throughout my energy field, several feet away from the body. I felt [it] in my heart. I felt inside as well—an instant connection that

154

again stunned me. "What is this coming into me?" And my reaction turned to a sorrow, and I apologized to this God for doubting and denying and being skeptical all these years. And then this appreciation consciousness that had been coming in changed into a compassion, a consoling.

Jeff has had many less dramatic experiences that he describes as clairsentience. On occasion he's had clairvoyant experiences, seeing images in the mind. He's also experienced clairaudience whereby he received an audible message through a disembodied voice. That unexpected visit came through a stranger. While it is difficult to put words to these experiences, Jeff is certain that his taiji was the gate opener for him, helping him release blockages in body, mind, and spirit. "I think that it's there for anybody to experience, but we have so much static and resistance that we build up in the course of our life here, in addition to just being in the physical form in the first place, that most of us don't experience that consciousness."

One of the summers that Chenoa worked for the National Parks Service, she was with a crew in Yosemite, clearing invasive species. The valley they were working in is an ancient Native American sacred site with petroglyphs still visible on the rock walls. The Natives, according to local history, were accused of stealing from the white people, so the cavalry came and basically exterminated the tribe. Deep in the mountains, this valley was a last hidden refuge.

As the crew worked to clear invasive non-native blackberries, one person was appointed fire tender to burn the cuttings. The fire pit was near the petroglyphs. As Chenoa took her turn, she practiced taiji between poking at and feeding it more brambles, she was open to the sense of having spirit company.

> I started hearing people walking towards the fire from all directions. Seeing movement, I turned and didn't see anybody. But I would see things out of the corner of my eye; I just couldn't see them straight on. I just had the feeling that they were all just curious, and open and accepting. It didn't feel like animosity or anything like that. It seemed like the fire was near all the places where they used to have their fires. Like it was their fire spot.

155

Others in the crew also had mystical experiences while tending that fire. Some people heard people yelling, and some heard what sounded like people making bird noises. Chenoa says, "I don't know if I would have noticed if I hadn't been doing taiji."

The Dissolution of Space and Time

> *The primal and temporal are originally not two: what makes the distinction is only temporal. When you discriminate, then action and stillness are not united, and primal energy becomes conditioned. When they are united, temporal energy is also primal, and there is no distinction between primal and temporal.*
>
> —The Secret of the Golden Flower (Cleary, 2000, p. 319)

When moments feel like hours, hours feel like minutes, or time simply disappears, the line from *Row, Row, Row Your Boat* takes on a different cast; because life, quite literally, becomes a dream. Despite the perception of time and space that living in the material world reinforces, the Buddhist, Vedic, and Sufi canons dismiss both as illusion. The Daoist point of view reduces space and time to part of the myriad things that arise from Dao:

> Space arises. Once there is space, there is qi; once there is qi, there is material existence; once there is material existence, there is a beginning; once there is a beginning, there is the passage of time—Heng Xian (Brindley et al., 2013).

Einstein, Godel, and their disciples in quantum physics—our high priests of modern scientific rationality—also claim there is no reality to time, backing up their assertations with theorems and formulas unfathomable to most of their congregation. Fortunately, Lynne McTaggart in her great distillation of quantum science explains,

156

Pure energy as it exists at the quantum level does not have time or space, but exists as a vast continuum of fluctuating charge. We, in a sense, are time and space. When we bring energy to conscious awareness through the act of perception, we create separate objects that exist in space through a measured continuum. By creating time and space, we create our own separateness (McTaggart, 2008, p. 174).

When taiji players begin to experience the elasticity of spacetime, it reflects a loosening of one's grip on a Newtonian measure of fixed, linear time and space, and acceptance of their interdependence. You can't have time without space, and you can't have space without time. Advanced players sometimes go a step further, learning to manipulate spacetime in push hands as if it were a viscous putty. Glimpses of this age-old koan emerge in little ways.

Witnessing a suspension of time, Rob realized that there was something internal missing from his martial arts. He was at a Passover Seder. His friend, a student of William C. C. Chen, pulled down a shade on a terrace door to screen the blinding light of the setting sun. Minutes later, the shade suddenly spun and popped off its hinges. It arced up in the air and was headed for the center of the dinner table. Without a break in his conversation, his hand floated up, caught the shade in midair and casually placed it on the table.

He never took his eyes off the person he was conversing with; he was never tense; he was not flustered. I was awestruck. What I just witnessed was the halting of time. We all pictured the certain devastation, but then time stood still, and the proverbial sword of Damocles was halted and neutralized in an amazingly efficient manner. Man, that was way cool. And that was when I thought, that's what I want to do ... learn how to stop time.

Lynn sometimes experiences a slowing of time reminiscent of her experience being on morphine after surgery. "During those times nothing was wrong. Nothing hurt. Everything is just right with the world."

These episodes transpire when she's totally relaxed. Three minutes will seem like two hours, and everything is great. Recently, she decided to take a break from painting in her studio.

> I came back and sat back down; I had written on my calendar when I had stopped. Seven minutes had gone by. But I did an hour's worth of things. I went and changed the laundry. I washed all these dishes in the sink. I went upstairs. I did something up there on the computer. Came back down. I don't know how that happened.

For Diana, the concept of time as an illusion came in very handy one morning during her morning commute. Habitually tardy to the office, she knew she was going to be about fifteen minutes late (again!). "After reading Master Jo's book and the whole idea about time, I just thought …okay 'If there's some kind of time warp thing where I'm going to be there on time, do it.'" Those fifteen minutes miraculously disappeared, and Diana arrived punctually at the office.

The slowing of time was a life saver for the premiere of a new music ensemble work for which Libby was playing oboe. There were about a dozen players, and the music was rhythmically intense, with jazzy syncopation and atonality that the ensemble was not grasping.

> Suddenly I had this sense that time slowed down. Everything slowed down, and instead of a rhythm that might have been quarter note=126 and dat dat bee pop, dad at, it was just really slow like quarter note=20. It was reminiscent of when you see slow motion photography, like a bullet going through space or being able to see a bee's wings move. This lasted for quite a while, and it was very helpful in terms of playing this music because instead of having a bit of a scramble and a little bit of a panic, it was just like dropping a stone in the water every 40 seconds.
>
> … the people around me started realizing that I was totally on with the rhythm. The conductor even said "Okay, just get into this groove like Libby's in. Just try

158

to get into that." And, of course, I was elated, I thought to myself this is the thing I'm going to be able to do for the rest of my life.

Still a relative beginner, Libby didn't connect the experience to taiji immediately, but a few days later her teacher, Steve Bennett, said as an aside, "I come from a lineage that can slow down time." Her jaw dropped. Today she remembers the episode not as euphoric, but one of total groundedness.

Stephe Watson experienced timelessness in the manner of the Sages—through extended meditation. After a period of feeling that his meditations were becoming a steeper and slipperier slope from which he might not know enough to come out of to sate his basic needs, he embarked on an extended retreat. He asked a nearby farmer to come check on him in three days and assumed the *santi* position from xingyi. He then took a day off and stood for another four days. He did not take scheduled breaks as one would in the safety of a retreat center or eat. He simply stood.

> I felt like I had the experience that people talk about of unending bliss or supreme bliss or that state. But I wouldn't have chosen those words. That was just sort of a reference. It felt like, at the most, bemusement. Afterwards, I could see why you would call it bliss. But, bliss, the term, feels relativistic. It seemed like a state beyond relativism.

In those three days, Stephe had no experience of monkey mind or discomfort. Had there not been the societal constraints to return to work Stephe thinks he could have continued standing indefinitely.

> Probably the biggest element of crossing the threshold was beginning it, because a moment before beginning, you're preparing. And then you do it and that is surrender. I don't know if surrender is exactly bliss. But it's a freedom. It's a freedom from your own consciousness.

Normally I want to have all of my motor forces directed by my consciousness. I want to examine my consciousness. Expand it, challenge it, compare it to others. I want to be in it and do with it all the time. So this is an experience of just surrendering consciousness.

Completely losing his sense of time, he also lost physical sensations including all physical awareness—whether it was day or night, cold or hot, wet by the night dew, being visited by bugs, or the deer that left tracks around him.

Steve Bennett specializes in Dim Mak, a martial technique utilizing the meridians and acupressure points, or cavities as he refers to them, to disarm an opponent. Given the deadly risk of these techniques, the practice is not widespread or very publicly offered for study. Bennett describes Ma Fun, a great praying mantis stylist, who was one of his teachers:

He had the capability of just using his fingertips and out of the blue tapping you on the eyes. His fingers were literally like some kind of feelers. The next thing you'd know it would be as if you'd been in an auto accident. You know how time stops and you count the hairs on the back of your wrists? ... Time would stop. ... when he hits the skin he goes deeper, when he hits the cavity, then he softens his wrist so he doesn't hurt you. That's the time stopping environment.

Bennett later found that Master Li Chung (also known as John Chung Li) was working on the same principles. This inspired Steve to begin to map the meridians and cavities that have this effect when struck or pressed.

By touching those cavities, says Bennett, you make your opponent fall down. "You stop their time, that's all. You don't go beyond that." Bennett says the martial tools for stopping time in push hands exist in all the taiji forms. He also recalls time stopping through deep visual connections. Practicing form is key to learning how to come in touch with the actual feeling of the cavities and meridian flows. "… people that take up residence in what I call Jiffyland; in quantum physics…. They pick up resonance in Jiffyland. Time is stopped for them all the time."

Space, of course, is an aspect of time, and time is measured by space. In physics this duality is unified—spacetime. In taiji, one works with space on many levels. In the form, one connects to the earth, heaven, and lateral dimensions. In a class, one can envelop the space incorporating the group or study the negative space bound by one's arms and torso. In push hands, control of the space between opponents is a basic premise.

Rick Barrett explains that in push hands space is a function and you have to be able to both create and collapse it even while it changes with your state of consciousness. One distinguishes between their own space, their opponent's space and shared space—three coexisting universes.

> If you have any one of those without the other, then you have an incomplete model. … Then my space, is what I happen to be focusing on at that time. Consequently, if I'm in a very fearful state my space collapses almost to one point. Basically, it's an implosion. You're collapsing your space and you're losing all sense of expansion.
>
> Whereas, the shared space is what you and I have created together. If we have big open space where we're both feeling relatively safe, then the space is allowed to expand. It can take up as much as we can put our attention on. Whereas, if you're pushing on me and you're collapsing my space, my space is shrinking, yours is getting bigger.

Martial arts training also emphasizes extending your awareness, says Rick. That intention to open space can extend infinitely. In meditation, you may instead collapse your space into one nondual point.

If you're collapsing your space, you're moving into a nondual state, in which there is no self, no other. There's only one point. A oneness. ...A true nondual state is no awareness of space. You're just now. When you start playing with space, then you've already separated into 'this not that.'

Maria was competing in a tournament in Chinatown, and as is often the case in the women's field, there was no one else in her division. The organizers found a couple of people from other divisions to push with her. In her second match, she was paired with a girl half her age, a kung fu student, who'd never played push hands.

At one point, she pushed; I yielded and somehow I neutralized, but it was like the floor moved. And we ended up in reverse positions. She was where I had been standing, I was where she had been standing, but neither of us had been pushed exactly. It was not like we even scored a point. We were in position. It was restricted hands and somehow we'd completely switched positions. And yet we were both so centered and nobody was off. I hadn't pushed her; she hadn't pushed me. We were just somehow rotated completely— instantaneously. The referee looked a little confused and called a point against me for moving. ...

That was an amazing feeling. And the thing is we were both connected, and we stayed connected. And neither one of us was off. We had just completely switched position.

Spacetime can, just like our physical senses, have parapsychological dimensions. Remote healing is an obvious example of this and quite common. By meditating and setting an intention, I can connect to individuals around the world, even if I haven't actually met them, to release pain or promote healing. Many paranormal healers work in the space around the body without actually touching it. Others barely touch the surface of the skin to effect a change deep within the fascia. Whether the space between us is five inches or five thousand miles really doesn't seem to make any difference. Form

162

and push hands practice train us to attune to connections through space and to dynamically interact with them, not as static objects, but intertwined relations.

As we've seen, the boundaries around all senses are virtually limitless to Stephe. In addition to the total surrender of consciousness that took away all sense of time and self, he has regular experiences with remote viewing and astral travel, and that has become a bit of a playground. Often, before traveling, especially if it is someplace he's not been to before, he'll visit nonphysically first. He'll experience elements of the place or have snapshots in his memory. When he actually arrives, it is an act of validation to verify relatively simple details like the color of a hotel room or placement of the furniture.

Synchronicity and Other Psychic Events

> *The light returns to the primal opening,*
> *So all psychic functions are calm.*
>
> —Secret of the Golden Flower (Cleary, 2000, p. 307)

> *If you have insight, says Chuang-tzu, "you use your*
> *inner eye, your inner ear, to pierce to the heart of things, and*
> *have no need of intellectual knowledge"* (Jung, 1960, p. 73).

In addition to growth in their psychic capabilities, many taiji players report greater awareness of synchronicities in their daily lives. Carl Jung, enamored by Daoist paradigms, found explanation there for the phenomena that his western philosophy could not explain, i.e. that by relaxing back into primal energy—before differentiation into "myriad things"—information simply appears (Jung, 1960, p. 70).

Synchronistic distortions of spacetime are a phenomenon that provided me a key clue that there is something greater out there than the worldview of my youth. In those days, a phone call from someone you were thinking about, or the fact that three out of five days a week my assistant at work and I showed up to the office wearing the same color earned a chuckle and was dismissed. But the more I did taiji, the more frequently I observed synchronicity.

163

Jung defined synchronicity as the "acausal connecting principal" or "a meaningful coincidence of two or more events," (Jung, 1960, p. 25). It is hard to know what he meant by meaningful as many synchronicities seem trivial to anyone except the observer[10]. For example, a common occurrence for me was the invasion of a new term on my horizon three times in as many days. Likewise, at work three people who didn't know each other offered similar ideas that steered a shift in my priorities or clarified a direction I needed to take on a project. Certainly they were meaningful in that they got my attention, but usually they were not important details.

However, as my taiji practice began to take on more supersensory qualities I felt like I was "absorbing the whole world" (Jung, 1960) or at least bizarrely connected pieces of it. Synchronicities thus became faith building markers. No matter how trivial they may seem, it feels as if it is the Dao's way of saying, are you listening? Are you paying attention? Are you being mindful enough in your activities to be able to witness the unfolding of consciousness that you experience? Are you staying open to the lessons being offered?

Those lessons often come in funny and inconsequential ways. Correspondence with a friend that discusses life issues is soon followed by a passage of a book providing guidance and perspective to guide response. Likewise, I regularly pick up books at random that hold the lesson needed to develop the line of inquiry I'm currently playing with. Or, out of the blue, I'll see or hear several references to the same book or person. The odd things I have in common with new acquaintances have led me to my closest friends and confidants.

Scheila sees synchronicity as a compass that teaches lessons on interrelatedness. For example, five different people told her she needed to study shamanism with a particular person. Then, through her connections, mention of a particular taiji teacher kept arising. One day, feeling a little crazy, she started to write down all the people she knew and discovered that all her networks are interrelated.

---

[10] Peter Kingsley posits that Jung's synchronicity was a politically correct label to mask his discomfort over the prophetic nature of his own precognitive visions and dreams (Kingsley, 2018, pp. 229–34).

In *Power Vs. Force: The Hidden Determinants of Human Behavior*, David Hawkins modernizes Jung's synchronicity. Modern physics demonstrates that what we are witnessing is actually simultaneity of events occurring in the universe. The connection between these events derives from neither cause and effect, gravity, nor magnetism. Rather, the connection occurs in the observer's consciousness.

> This relationship is a concept in the mind of the observer; it isn't necessary that any corollary external event exist in the universe. Unless there's an underlying attractor pattern, nothing can be experienced. Thus, the entire manifest universe is its own simultaneous expression and experience of itself (Hawkins, 2002, p. 134).

Visions of Good and Evil

Taiji players often report more frequent observation of other psychic events as well, including precognition, dreams, spirits, and visions. After Eleanor started taking a seniors' taiji class, such events quickly became quite commonplace. She recounts a vision a few days after her taiji instructor's wife opened a tattoo shop.

> I was lying on my couch and all of a sudden they showed me a bear. They showed me a Native Indian motif, and I know nobody in my family or friends with tattoos. So when I came in, I said to [my teacher], "Bruce, that must be for your wife." And I told him what I saw. He said, "That is actually my wife's store. Making Indian motifs."

Another day, sitting in her easy chair watching the psychic John Edwards on television, she suddenly saw a beautiful baby all in white. Five minutes later, her niece called from San Francisco to tell her about the birth of her grandson. The niece confirmed that everything around the baby was white.

Eleanor's frequent visions include spirits of dead relatives, usually her mother, appearing in crowds on television or visiting her while she is cooking dinner.

> They can show you anything you want. They can show you a life come through. They show me life. They also show me bad things. They showed me when my husband needed to come out of a [seizure] in such a way that I could get help from the hospital staff to save his life.

Eleanor's visions also include what she calls dark spirits that she works hard to keep away. Flooded with such information as Eleanor is, it is valuable to maintain the Daoist perspective toward evil. Heguanzi, the third-century-BCE, so-called Peasant Cap Master, wrote,

> Good and evil are mutually defining,
> their mandate is called the return cycle.
> When things reach extremes they revert,
> their mandate is called circular flow.
> (Wells, 2013, pp. 111–13)

Modern master, Waysun Liao, elaborates on evil as part of the yin yang continuum. Energies, he says, moving toward the centerpoint, Dao—or God—are creative forces moving in the direction of life (yang). Destructive energies are moving away from Dao (yin). Despite the emotional bite of the word evil, it is necessary:

> In God's universe nothing is wasted. Everything has a purpose and a job to do at whatever stage of the journey it's in. Evil has a purpose and a job too...
>
> When you see lions go out to kill and eat, they're just doing their job. Bacteria eating away at dead tissue are just doing their job. Predators and scavengers are very necessary in nature. Without them, our planet would be a mess. You cannot say bacteria or lions are "evil." They're just doing

their job. We are the ones that turn our noses up at what they do and label it as "evil."

That destructive side of power is equal to the nourishing power in our universe. Remember how we said the sun couldn't function if it didn't have both gravity pulling in and heat and light radiating out? Balance requires both sides of the coin. That includes the nourishing and destructive power of our universe (Liao, 2010, pp. 64–6).

For some, like Eleanor, visions and dreams may be uninhibited reflections of the subconscious at a level where the ego is still in play. They may be a precognitive or psychic nondual view of reality, but they may also be tinged with details of the subconscious. Lawrence LeShan explains:

The fact that "evil entities" are frequently reported to be encountered in spiritual work is not surprising ... As has been shown in many mystical training groups (as well as psychotherapeutic experience) inner growth and change—particularly if done at a rapid rate—bring to the surface of consciousness some not-so-lovely parts of ourselves. If these are not understood as coming from inside ourselves they are likely to be projected outward on others or as evil forces and entities (LeShan, 2003, p. 193).

More simply, Livia Kohn writes:

[T]he more out of tune any individual (including plants, animals, and ghosts) is, the more "evil" he is from the point of Dao, the more unhappy he feels, the less fortunate he appears. Such "evil" is not fundamental; it is not rooted in the cosmos. It is merely a deviation, a change in pattern, it is a different wavelength, an unmatched pitch... (Kohn, 2016, pp. 23–4).

Recognition of a vision's subconscious nature may only be

possible in hindsight, but is an important aspect of one's personal growth. To create space for such self-awareness and to allow it to guide one's interpretation of neurosis and fears that take on mind forms, such as evil spirits, is a step toward greater consciousness. That, in turn, facilitates one's ability to stay with the middle way, aligned with Dao, responding to thoughts or events with mindfulness. Primary reality acknowledges all natural energies as projections emanating from source as myriad things. In verse 60 of the *Dao De Jing*, Laozi advises:

> Rule a big country
> the way you cook a small fish.
> If you keep control by following the Way,
> troubled spirits won't act up.
> They won't lose their immaterial strength,
> but they won't harm people with it,
> nor will wise souls come to harm.
> And so, neither harming the other,
> these powers will come together in unity.
>
> —Laozi (Le Guin, 1998, p. 78)

In the twelfth-century text, *Immortal Sisters*, Sun Bu-er and her twentieth-century commentator, Chen Yingning, again caution practitioners not to get too distracted by events like visions of the worldly nature:

> The Womb Breath ...
>
> If you want the elixir to form quickly,
> First get rid of illusory states.
> Attentively guard the spiritual medicine;
> With every breath return to the beginning of the creative.
> The energy returns, coursing through the three islands;
> The spirit, forgetting, unites with the ultimate.
> Coming this way and going this way.

No place is not truly so.

Commentary by Chen Yingning:

… Actually, "illusory states" are hallucinations produced by hidden influences in the body under certain circumstances. Sometimes they attract and charm people, sometimes they frighten people, sometimes they anger people, sometimes they sadden people; they may induce people to mistake them for spiritual communications or powers, and they may induce people to enter false paths. In extreme cases they can cause dementia and self-destruction. People may have chance visions or hear voices, and claim they have met the saints.

Things like this are all illusory states, or they might be called illusory objects; they should be swept away. Without objective perception, it is hard to distinguish them from reality. That is why learners need to follow teachers. There are people who have studied Taoism for decades without negative influences presenting obstacles, all because they have not really practiced the Tao.

… The Old Master Lao-tzu said, "Returning to the root is called quietude; quietude is called going back to Life." This is the meaning of energy returning. The human body originally comes from the great void; once it falls into material form, it has resistance, and cannot merge with the great void. Only those imbued with the Tao can forget all material form. Once material form is removed from the focus of attention, then one merges with the great void (Cleary, 2000, pp. 434–5).

Tim did just that after a particularly potent qigong class that involved an eye exercise. Turning the eyes in the sockets and looking in unusual directions, he experienced a loss of equilibrium and found that things around him were shaking.

I felt what started to feel like a numbing sensation in my feet, and I played with the idea that maybe that's what rooting felt closer to being. So I just let that go and found that my feet were more connected to the ground and sensations of energy coming up through the ground... really felt like it was glossing over all the internal organs in my body.

That night with one of his friends he discussed the concept of surrender as seen in the opening of the form.

I found it incredibly difficult to do in the class. But in this experience, my friend and I were discussing some things that were making me unhappy, and we were discussing just letting go. And then we did.

Rising up out of our bodies, not looking down like in a death sequence like you'd see on TV, but actually rising straight up and being able to see things on all sides. And we rose up into a plane that was just light or energy, not necessarily bright, but it was all encompassing and ... it was a really amazing feeling and we were pretty much One in that plane.

The act of perception is a filtering of energies through our physical and egoic forms, while struggle against the flow leads to suffering. The fact that people have out of body experiences and visions, and access lessons from them, is a sign of openness to higher level consciousness. It is akin to feeling the buzz in my hands as I hold a qi ball; it is a perception of a higher level of energy filtered through sense and experience—a step on the path toward the prime reality energy of nonduality, where all is unified in the pregnant stillness prior to distinctions between yin/yang, good/bad, you/me that become possible with complete surrender.

Through the Looking Glass:
Achieving Personal Spiritual Mastery

You sit and listen to the stringless tune, you clearly understand the mechanism of creation.

When your work reaches here, you hear the sound of the music of the immortals, and there are also the tones of bells and drums. The five energies assemble at the source, the three flowers gather on the peak; that means the true sense of real knowledge of the true essence of consciousness is present in the will, and the vitality, energy, and spirit have been refined and united. It is a state like when a raven comes to roost in the evening. The mind field is open and clear, knowledge and wisdom spontaneously grow, and one clearly understands the writings of the three teachings, tacitly realizes one's roots in former lives, foreknows what bodes good and ill for the future; the whole world is as though in one's palm. You see for myriad miles and have the subtle psychic faculties available to complete human beings. This is real being.

—Commentary on Ancestor Lü by Chang San-Feng
(Cleary, 2000, p. 192)

O nly the rarified few in any spiritual practice attain full blown spiritual enlightenment and the wisdom of its moment to moment awareness. Nevertheless, many taiji players, even the less than sparkling ones, recognize the practice as a process, providing a consistent platform in which at least occasionally one grows. The art is so full of intellectual, physical, and metaphysical details, that it is a bit like peeling an onion. There is always another layer from which to look at a move, and each understanding changes the whole experience, renewing beginner's joy, and staving off

171

boredom. Any methodology for spiritual development embedded into taiji practice is indistinguishable from methodology to develop the body and heart mind. Each posture contains relationships between yin and yang, substantial and insubstantial, and the five elements. The five elements, of course, encompass aspects of the human experience—from organs of the body, emotions, senses, and heavenly directions—but that is categorization and has little to do with how one experiences the divine. Spiritual manifestations can develop concurrently with the mind or body, or not, depending on what the practitioner is ready for and open to.

Cheng Man Ching instructed his students to focus on form, quieting the mind first and then allowing other aspects to organically develop.

> Secure mind and ch'i in the dantien. ... This is the meaning of "seek the release of the mind" and "is the host at home." After a long time, the ch'i naturally passes through the coccyx, spreads along the backbone, and travels up through the occipital region to the top of the head. Then it descends to the dantien. This is the unification of the jen and tu meridians and the coupling of the heart and kidney. You cannot, however, attain this after practicing just a short while. More importantly, you cannot force it! It must be completely natural. If you do attain it your T'ai Chi Ch'uan has the potential to reach the highest level where your spirit will become immortal. Longevity and good health will be your lot (Cheng, 1985, pp. 41–2).

Understanding taiji as an approach to life, Chris incorporates what is also a primary tenet of Zen, taking in each moment as it arises. In the margins between the realms of mind and spirit, Eastern teachings encourage process rather than outcomes as a path to understanding the underlying impermanence of our seemingly objective world. Attention to a process such as walking—the feel of your feet touching the ground, the wind in your hair, the smell of the air—is far more important than reaching a destination. To be aware, moment by moment, and totally present to that moment, is the goal of all nondual spiritual practices. Taiji, through physical movement, trains us to slow down and be mindful. In form and push hands practice one plays in the space between movements. There one finds time to listen, read reactions and responses, and observe what arises with another person in the mix. Consistent and repetitive acts of slowing down, breathing, rooting, and interacting begin to permeate one's being, leaking into one's general demeanor, one's approach to the workday, artistic endeavors, and world view.

Slowing down his form to focus on the stages between things really struck a chord, says Chris.

> One of the things I like to do when I'm vacationing is right when you get to your destination, turn around and start heading back because the destination is just a place to stop for the night and take a shower. It's all about the journey for me; and one of the reasons why I like the concept of taiji is because I tend to be looking in the spaces between things.

The simple step by step experience of the journey as it is, is a beautiful acceptance of Now. At any level of skill this attainment is observable, and reward is not reserved for the master. Mere mortals are quite likely to experience at least occasional precious moments, and the taiji form provides a training platform for that.

After some five decades of practice, Maggie Newman and Ken Van Sickle consistently demonstrate beginner's joy at the slightest details of a weight shift or slight neutralizing turn. That kind of discipline and attention is a bridge to taiji as spiritual practice. Staying grounded in the details of the physical body can create a platform of safety from which mystical moments emerge, a contemplative platform from which to reassess one's perspective toward life. This *zhen*, or flow state, is when a *wu wei* moment of effortless action reveals itself.

This state of complete moment to moment consciousness unfettered by self-preference—William James' sciousness—is seen in peak performance athletes. Witness Michael Phelps' Olympic brilliance, Rodger Federer's tennis, or Michael Jordan's years of other worldliness on the court. They all appear calm and unemotional as they systematically dismantle their competitors wearing the equanimity of *wu wei*. Martial artists, musicians, artists, writers, and gardeners all describe a shifting sense of self and time during effortless immersion, while feelings of action flow through them.

Often called a moving meditation, form, push hands, or qigong practice readily trigger this feeling of spiritual connectedness as well.

Diana's evolution was one of spiritual as well as personal expansion. Despite being raised to go to church every Sunday, she no longer had any formal religious practice. When she practiced taiji, especially outdoors, she would find herself praying. "It was like a meditation; it just came from doing it. I didn't plan to do it. It just came with doing it. It's your connection to spirit and the force—the energetic life force."

In order to advance in push hands, one must learn to listen, feel, and respond to a partner's energy. Advanced players break down their sense of self and solidity and can merge with another's energy. Moving past the discomfort of fear and intimacy, that dissolution of sense of self leads to some profound moments.

Scheila developed the personal paradigm,

As above so below, as within so without. There is no separation. I'm not saying I'm doing it every moment. My intention is to bring myself back and be very conscious of the weaving of nonseparation. And when I get knocked off my pins, I come back, and I say to myself: It started out with what is truth. And so I sift it on down, and it comes to this … You are me, and I am you. There's no separation.

Taiji helped Luke think about the world, his life, and his place in it.

I was exposed at an early age to nature and all the creatures in it, the other little people and big people that inhabit it—from bees to deer. So on that level things happen without words. … I keep an open mind because language is

174

metaphorical. Every word is a metaphor. There's so much talking in the world because metaphors have to be balanced.

Then I realized after a while that if there is a God, God is the ground, which is beyond metaphor. Shut up and God will speak to you—but in a nonmetaphorical way. God speaks to me; the evidence is right there. It is in every tree that's growing and every leaf, every butterfly, every fly, mosquito, slug, spider, every cat, every squirrel, birds. These are all the world of God.

Carole points out that in Christianity, Judaism, Islam, Hinduism, and even pagan religions, it's important for people to put names on things and create structures around them.

But taiji's not constructed. In fact, it's letting go of all that stuff—moving outside of the construct. … I've been seeing for a long time that people need structures. They help us in many ways. But I've always had trouble clinging to them, and so taiji helps me to see that. You let go of them. You still exist. You don't need those belief structures. Taiji has helped me along that path, but it's not the first door that opened. There are a lot of doors on this hallway.

Linda describes a shift, from trying to be happy to feeling much more like part of the life force on the planet. Leaving behind a life with an intellectual approach to things, accompanied by chronic headaches and the incumbent pain relievers, she shed depression.

Now the best parts of my days touch everything around me. So it's a very different feeling energywise. … In some ways I feel younger than I did ten years ago because I feel lighter in many ways. I feel less of my mind intellectually worrying, wondering about things and more willing to understand that I'm able to do what I feel I need to do.

When people play taiji for a long time, says David Chandler, their sense of personal power is transformed. They don't have to prove anything and have the confidence to just be with another person. They also have the confidence to be extraordinarily generous. Having witnessed a number of Chinese masters who demonstrated "having steel inside the cotton," David believes that you have to go deep in your stance to achieve this level of personal development.

When you experience that deep place for yourself, physically, and you experience nature with no filters, you begin to touch that place within yourself. You open because you're experiencing extreme kindness. Witnessing an act of extreme kindness and extreme generosity—then that's going to trigger the same within yourself [but] towards others. It's a trigger for more people to have that experience, and it gets passed on.

One day while living in New York City, David finished his taiji practice. All of a sudden he felt as if his spine unzipped and his body opened.

It was as if the universe, a handful of stars, reached into my body, and my body was like a puppet. It wiggled me around and was dancing me. It was like the universe, the Dao, took over the movement of my body. I was filled with stars, and I witnessed this exquisite sense of oneness with everything. No separation except there was this puppet that was my body. And I felt this back up into the endless open space, filled with stars. And this changed me.

Having witnessed others' journeys to mystical realms, David notices that the fear of not coming back can trigger terror. Sometimes that is fear of not returning; sometimes it is because it is so awesome.

It changes you because you want it to happen every day. It's that silver box experience. So you go back to your taiji, and say "and again?" Every day is different. You don't step in the same river twice. It's always a new river. You step there, but the river's gone by. So that experience has been by, and it's been through you. Now you're onto the next layer where something else will happen. And that's, I think, one of the great teachings of taiji. What's next? What's next? You're always in the now. And that's when all time exists.

As David says, opening to the divine is not always a comfortable process. Tom D. found his way to taiji looking for guidance. He was practicing pranayama breathing exercises and kundalini meditation out of a book and realized he was experiencing "kundalini psychosis." He elected to not pursue esoteric practices without a teacher, out of both fear and respect.

> Certainly there is more than meets the eye. That has been made clear to me… Taiji opened up the world of my spiritual life to me. And I have spent my life trying to embrace that and integrate it with my mental and physical existence.

Don Miller also recalls experiences of destabilizing levels of higher consciousness before he developed root. He came to understand through his study of the Daoist spiritual methods that with deeper root you can explore and assume altered states of consciousness in a safer way. By developing root, and working on lower chakras, then you can open the upper chakras without becoming spacy. Root enables you to maintain your alignment and position between heaven and earth. This balance and connection to earth—that root the Daoists are explicit about—is a foundation for Don's meditation and spiritual work.

A kundalini crisis further affirmed Don's faith in root. Seven years into his own practice, he saw his cousin walking down Mass Ave. in Cambridge. He had so much energy shooting up to the top of his head that his eyes were blazing like laser beams. People on the street would catch his eye and turn away. He looked like a crazy man, and, in fact, he was profoundly disturbed. Don was able to work with him on grounding and rooting. "It saved his ass. Within a couple of sessions he was able to calm down and was able to absorb some of this energy without going nuts. That confirmed to me that I was on the right track in terms of which is the horse and which is the cart," said Don.

As these accounts attempt to demonstrate, it doesn't matter where you are when you start or how good a martial artist you become. With diligence and good teachers, the practice of taiji can be spiritually transformative. For many, attention to martial application drives progress, while others are content to enjoy the buzz of a floating form. It is my hope that this offering adds a little understanding and perspective as the nondual world reveals itself to us.

My teacher, Maggie Newman, liked to remind us from time to time that, "Words don't cook the rice." May we let go of ideas and intentions, fears and fantasies, paradigms and principles, and simply practice.

Glossary

bagua – Daoist eight trigrams motif or energy map, martial art based on circular patterns intended to defend the eight directions

chakras – Sanskrit word for 7 energy centers in the body

Dao, also **Tao**, – The way, underlying principles governing the universe

daoyin – healing exercises, precursor to qigong

dim mak – branch of marital arts that targets points on the meridians to disable opponents

fa jin – an explosive discharge of energy

golden elixir – described by Mantak Chia as a mixture of saliva with hormones and qi that has extreme healing qualities

ichuan – standing meditation postures

jing – a person's highest essence

koan – a paradoxical question or riddle, used in Zen Buddhism todemonstrate the inadequacy of logical reasoning and to provoke enlightenment

kundalini – term from a style of yoga denoting energy coiled at the base of the spine, style of yoga directed toward releasing energy from the base of the spine

Laozi, also known as Lao Tzu, Laotzu – sixth-century-BCE sage credited with writing the *Dao De Jing*

li – movement of the body

meridians – pathways through the body associated with organs along which vital energy flow, used in Chinese medicine

neidan – meditation practices that foster internal alchemy

neigong – energy gathering exercises, meditation

nonduality – spiritual concept of oneness, unity

peng – expansive energy used in ward off move in taiji forms

qi – lifeforce energy

qigong – modern term for healing exercises, literally qi work or energy work

root – relationship or connection of the body to the ground and gravity

sciousness – consciousness without sense of self, term coined by William James

shen – spirit

song – relaxation of the body and mind

shen – pure mind, spirit

taijiquan – style of martial arts, distinguished by slow movements, internal energy and Daoist history

te – inner power, integrity

tui na – massage/body work informed by meridian theory

tui shou – push hands, two person exercises

wu – emptiness, nothing, void

wuji – the infinite

wu wei – movement without doing, action through nonaction

xin – heart mind

xingyi – an internal martial art characterized by linear movements

yi, also **i** – intent, consciousness

yang – expansive energy, associated with masculinity, strength, brightness, et. al

yin – retreating energy, associated with femininity, softness, darkness, etc.

yin yang – Daoist concept of duality

Zuangzi, also known as **Chuang Tzu**, fourth-century-BCE philosopher and writer

Bibliography

Abram, D. (1996) The Spell of the Sensuous, (New York: Vintage Books).

Acocella, J. (2007) *The Diary of Vaslav Nijinsky,* (Urbana: University of Illinois Press).

Astin, J., Shapiro, S., Eisenberg, D. & Forys, K. (2003) "Mind-body Medicine: State of the Science, Implications for Practice." *The Journal of the American Board of Family Practice,* 16, 131-47.

Barnes, P.M., Bloom, B. & Nahin, R.L. (2008) "Complementary and alternative medicine use among adults and children: United States, 2007." *Natl Health Stat Report,* 1-23.

Barrett, R. (2005) *Taijiquan: Through the Western Gate,* (Berkeley: Blue Snake Books).

Bennell, K. & Hinman, R. (2011) "A Review of the Clinical Evidence for Exercise in Osteoarthritis of the Hip and Knee." *Journal of Science and Medicine in Sport,* 14, 4-9.

Brennan, B.A. (1987) Hands of Light: A Guide to Healing Through the Human Energy Field, (New York: Bantam Books).

Bricklin, J. (2007) *Sciousness,* (Guilford, CT: Eirini Press).

Bricklin, J. (2016) *Illusion of Will, Self, and Time,* (Albany: State University of New York Press).

Brindley, E.F., Goldin, P.R. & Klein, E.S. (2013) "A Philosophical Translation of the Heng Xian." *Dao,* 12, 145-51.

Chang, D.S.T. (1986) The Complete System of Self-Healing Internal Exercises, (San Francisco: Tao Publishing).

Chen, K.W. (2004) "An Analytic Review of Studies on Measuring Effects of External Qi in China." *Alternative Therapies, Health and Medicine,* 10, 38-50.

Cheng, M.C. *A poem by Prof. Cheng Man Ching* [Online]. Taiji Forum. Available: https://taiji-forum.com/tai-chi-taiji/tai-chi-philosophy/poem-prof-cheng-man-ching/ [Accessed 2017].

Cheng, M.C. (1985) Cheng Tzu's Thirteen Treatises on T'ai Chi Ch'uan, (North Atlantic Books).

Cleary, T. (1991) Understanding the Mysteries: Further Teachings of Lao-tzu, (Boston: Shambhala).

Cleary, T. (1999) "The Book of Balance and Harmony." *The Taoist Classics: The Collected Translations of Thomas Cleary Volume 2.* (Boston: Shambhala).

Cleary, T. (2000) "Immortal Sisters: Secrets of Taoist Women." *The Taoist Classics: The Collected Translations of Thomas Cleary Volume 3.* (Boston: Shambhala).

Cohen, K.S. (1997) The Way of Qigong: The Art and Science of Chinese Energy Healing, (New York: Ballantine Books).

Deng, M.-D. (1993) Chronicles of Tao: The Secret Life of a Taoist Master, (San Francisco: Harper).

Dong, P. & Raffill, T. (2006) Empty Force: The Power of Chi for Self-Defense and Energy Healing, (Berkeley: Blue Snake Books).

Emerson, R.W. (2003) *Nature and Other Writings,* (Boston: Shambhala).

Gajdosova, K. "Undifferentiated as a Source of Independence and Authority." Authority vs. Authenticity: International Conference on Daoist Studies, 2018 Beijing Normal University.

Gajdosova, K. (10 June 2019) *RE: Immortality and Eternalism.* [Personal Communication].

Gardner, H. (2008) Multiple Intelligences: New Horizons in Theory and Practice, (Perseus Books Group).

Grof, S. & Bennett, H.Z. (1993) The Holotropic Mind - The Three Levels of Human Consciousness and How They Shape Our Lives, (New York: Harper Collins).

Hall, A., Maher, C., Latimer, J. & Ferreira, M. (2009) "The Effectiveness of Tai Chi for Chronic Musculoskeletal Pain Conditions: A Systematic Review and Meta-analysis." *Arthritis and Rheumatology,* 61, 717-24.

Hawkins, D.R. (2002) Power Vs. Force: The Hidden Determinants of Human Behavior, (Carlsbad: Hayhouse).

Hinton, D. (2016) *Existence: A Story,* (Boulder: Shambhala).

Ho, C. (2018) *Internal Alchemy for Everyone,* (St. Petersburg, FL: Three Pines Press).

Hoffman, E. *Awakening of Kundalini* [Online]. New Brain—New World. Available: www.newbrainneworld.com. [Accessed 2007].

Iwamoto, J., Sato, Y., Takeda, T. & Matsumoto, H. (2010) "Effectiveness of Exercise in the Treatment of Lumbar Spinal Stenosis, Knee Osteoarthritis, and Osteoporosis." *Aging Clinical and Experimental Research, 22,* 116-22.

James, W. (1890) *Principles of Psychology,* (New York: Henry Holt).

James, W. (1897) "Address by the President." *Proceedings of the Society for Psychical Research, 12,* 5.

James, W. (1900) "On a Certain Blindness in Human Beings." *Talks to Teachers on Psychology: And to Students on Some of Life's Ideals.* (New York: Henry Holt).

James, W. (1902) The Varieties of Religious Experience: A Study in Human Nature, (New York: Barnes and Noble Classics).

James, W. (1910) "A Suggestion about Mysticism." *Journal of Philosophy, Psychology, and Scientific Methods, 7,* 85-92.

Johnson, W. (1996) The Posture of Meditation: A Practical Manual for Meditators of All Traditions, (Boston: Shambhala).

Jung, C. (1960) *Synchronicity: An Acausal Connecting Principle,* (Princeton: Princeton University Press).

Kaiguo, C. & Shunchao, Z. (1996) *Opening the Dragon Gate: The Making of a Modern Taoist Wizard,* (Tokyo, Rutland, Vermont, Singapore: Tuttle Publishing).

Kalweit, H. (1988) Dreamtime and Inner Space: The World of the Shaman, (Boston and London: Shambhala).

Kaptchuk, T. (1983) *The Web That Has No Weaver,* (Chicago: Congdon and Weed).

Keeney, B. (2007) Shaking Medicine: The Healing Power of Ecstatic Movement, (Rochester, VT: Destiny Books).

Kingsley, P. (2018) *Catafalque: Carl Jung and the End of Humanity,* (London: Catafalque Press).

Kit, W.K. (2019) *Taijiquan Treatise of Zhang San Feng!* [Online]. Available:http://shaolin.org/video-clips-7/wudang-taijiquan/treatise/treatise01.html [Accessed 2019].

Kohn, L. (2010) Sitting In Oblivion: The Heart of Daoist Meditation, (Dunedin, FL: Three Pines Press).

Kohn, L. (2011) "Mental Health in Daoism and Modern Science." *In:* Kohn, L. (ed.) *Living Authentically: Daoist Contributions to Modern Psychology.* (St. Petersburg, FL: Three Pines Press).

Kohn, L. (2012) *A Source Book in Longevity,* (St. Petersburg, FL: Three Pines Press).

Kohn, L. (2016) Science and the Dao: From the Big Bang to Lived Perfection, (St. Petersburg, FL: Three Pines Press).

Kohn, L. (2017) *Pristine Affluence: Daoist Roots in the Stone Age,* (St. Petersburg, FL: Three Pines Press).

Lauche, R., Langhorst, J., Dobos, G. & Cramer, H. (2013) "A Systematic Review and Meta-analysis of Tai Chi for Osteoarthritis of the Knee." *Complementary Therapies in Medicine,* 21, 396-406.

Le Blanc, C. (1985) *Huainanzi* [Online]. In Wikipedia. Available: https://en.wikipedia.org/wiki/Huainanzi#CITEREFLe_Blanc1993 [Accessed 2018].

Le Guin, U. (1998) Tao Te Ching - A Book about the Way and the Power of the Way, (Boston & London: Shambhala).

Lee, M.S., Pittler, M.H. & Ernst, E. (2007) "Tai chi for rheumatoid arthritis: systematic review." *Rheumatology,* 46, 1648-51.

Leshan, L. (2003) The Medium, the Mystic, and the Physicist: Toward a General Theory of the Paranormal, (New York: Allworth Press).

Leshan, L. (2011) [Personal Communication].

Leshan, L. (2012) *Landscapes of the Mind: The Faces of Reality,* (Guilford, CT: Eirini Press).

Liao, W. (2010) *Tao: The Way of God,* (Oak Park, IL: Taichi Tao Productions).

Liping, W. (2019) *Daoist Internal Mastery*, (Three Pines Press).

Lipton, B. (2005) *The Biology of Belief,* (Santa Rosa: Mountain of Love/Elite Books).

Liu, D. (1986) *T'ai Chi Ch'uan & Meditation,* (New York: Schocken Books).

Loy, D. (1985) "Wei-wu-wei: Nondual Action." *Philosophy East and West,* Vol. 35, 73.

Ma, J. (1988) "Mechanism of qigong - magnetic resonance." First World Conference for Academic Exchange of Medical Qigong.

McTaggart, L. (2008) The Field: The quest for the secret force of the universe, (New York: Harper).

Mitchell, S. (1999) *Dao de Jing: An Illustrated Journey,* (New York: HarperCollins Publishers).

Pearce, J.C. (2002) The Biology of Transcendence - A Blueprint of the Human Spirit, (Rochester, VT: Park Street Press).

Phillips, S.P. (2019) Tai Chi, Baguazhang and the Golden Elixir: Internal Martial Arts Before the Boxer Uprising, (Louisville, CO: Angry Baby Books).

Radin, D., Schlitz, M. & Baur, C. (2015) "Distant Healing Intention Therapies: An Overview of the Scientific Evidence." *Global advances in health and medicine,* 4, 67-71.

Reid, M.C., Papaleontiou, M., Ong, A., Breckman, R., Wethington, E. & Pillemer, K. (2008) "Self-management Strategies to Reduce Pain and Improve Function Among Older Adults in Community Settings: A Review of the Evidence." *Pain Medicine,* 9, 409-24.

Rodgers, J. & Ruff, W. 2003. *Harmony of the World.* Killen, AL: Kepler Label.

Rose, K. (2007) "What is Qi?" Qi The Journal of Traditional Easter Health & Fitness, 17, 20-7.

Roth, H.D. (1999) Original Tao: Inward Training (Nei-yeh) and the Foundations of Taoist Mysticism, (New York: Columbia University Press).

Schieir, O., Adeponle, A., Milette, K. & Thombs, B.D. (2010) "Efficacy of Tai Chi for Chronic Musculoskeletal Pain Conditions: Is the Evidence Ready for Meta-analysis? Comment on the Article by Hall et al." *Arthritis Care Research,* 62, 139-40.

Schwartz, S.A. (2017) "The Manipulation of Perceived Reality Through Nonlocal Intention." *Explore,* 13, 12-5.

Slingerland, E. (2003) Effortless Action: Wu-wei as Conceptual Metaphor and Spiritual Ideal in Early China, (New York: Oxford University Press).

Smithsonian (1996) *Egyptian Mummies* [Online]. Available: http://www.si.edu/Encyclopedia_SI/nmnh/mummies.htm [Accessed].

Stanley-Baker, M. (2012) "Palpable Access to the Divine: Daoist Medieval Massage, Visualisation and Internal Sensation." *Asian Medicine,* 7, 101-27.

Star, J. (2003) Tao Te Ching: The Definitive Edition, (New York: Tarcher).

Trumble, W.R., Stevenson, A. & Brown, L. (2002) *Shorter Oxford English dictionary on historical principles,* (New York: Oxford University Press).

Wang, H. "Intention and Sympathetic Resonance in Daoist Practice." Authority vs. Authenticity: International Conference on Daoist Studies, 2018 Beijing Normal University.).

Watson, B. (2003) *Zhuangzi: Basic Writings,* (New York: Columbia University Press).

Wayne, P.M. & Fuerst, M. (2013) The Harvard Medical School Guide to Tai Chi: 12 Weeks to a Healthy Body, Strong Heart, and Sharp Mind, (Boston: Shambhala).

Webster, M. *Merriam Webster Dictionary* [Online]. Available: m-w.com [Accessed 2016].

Wells, M. (2005) Scholar Boxer: Cháng Naizhou's Theory of Internal Martial Arts and the Evolution of Taijiquan, (Berkeley: Blue Snake Books).

Wells, M. (2013) The Pheasant Cap Master and the End of History: Linking Religion to Philosophy in Early China, (St. Petersburg, FL: Three Pines Press).

Wikipedia. (2016) *Abraham Abulafia* [Online]. In Wikipedia. [Accessed 2016]

Wikipedia. (2019) *Alexandre-Émile Béguyer de Chancourtois* [Online]. In Wikipedia. [Accessed 2019].

Wolinsky, S.P.D. (1999) *The Way of the Human: The Quantum Psychology Notebooks,* (Capitola, California: Quantum Institute).

Wong, E. (2000) The Tao of Health, Longevity, and Immortality - the Teachings of Immortals Chung and Lü, (Boston & London: Shambhala).

Yan, J.H., Gu, W.J., Sun, J., Zhang, W.X., Li, B.W. & Pan, L. (2013) "Efficacy of Tai Chi on Pain, Stiffness and Function in Patients with Osteoarthritis: A Meta-analysis." *PLoS One,* **8,** e61672.

Author Bio – Denise L. Meyer

Denise Meyer started studying taiji over twenty years ago, first with world push hands champion Stephen Watson, then with Cheng Man Ching's senior student, Maggie Newman. She has also been heavily influenced by work with Rick Barrett, Ken Van Sickle, Robert Mann and Wei-Ming Chen. A classical saxophonist by training (Northwestern University) and founder and publisher of a boutique press (Eirini Press) focusing on non-duality, she has published books by Lawrence LeShan, Jonathan Bricklin, and others. She has worked in public relations and communications as an independent consultant and at Yale University. By day, she is currently the web content editor and technical specialist at the Yale School of Public Health.

Starting as a quintessentially typical practitioner of taiji, Meyer, like many advancing players, quickly realized that there was a lot more going on in this practice than first meets the eye. Her book, *Swimming in the Sea of Qi: The Taiji Path to Energetic and Spiritual Awareness*, demonstrates and adds meaning to seemingly mundane manifestations of qi to create context for the western practitioner.

Her talk at the 2018 International Daoist Conference in Beijing was published in the *Journal of Daoist Studies* (edited by Livia Kohn, PhD). She led a 2-hour workshop exploring space at the 2019 International Daoist Conference in Los Angeles. She has been certified to teach in the Cheng Man Ching lineage by Maggie Newman and Ken Van Sickle.

www.ingramcontent.com/pod-product-compliance
Lightning Source LLC
Chambersburg PA
CBHW030513100426
42813CB00001B/29